PUPPETRY FOR MENTALLY HANDICAPPED PEOPLE

HUMAN HORIZONS SERIES

PUPPETRY FOR MENTALLY HANDICAPPED PEOPLE

Caroline Astell-Burt

A CONDOR BOOK
SOUVENIR PRESS (E & A) LTD

ISBN 0 285 64932 9 casebound
ISBN 0 285 64933 7 paperback

Printed in Great Britain by
Ebenezer Baylis & Son Ltd
The Trinity Press, Worcester, and London

To Warwick

Contents

Acknowledgments

The author owes grateful thanks to the staff and children of Dr Barnardo's Ian Tetley School for the early opportunities given to me while I was a house-parent there;

Colin Lee from the Harrogate College of Arts and Adult Studies for his valuable encouragement right at the very beginning;

Mencap, Yorkshire and Humberside Region, Mike Brown, Ken Pugh and their staff;

The Geoffrey Ost Award Committee, Sheffield University;

Dr Trevor Wright for the valuable research I was able to do at the Ryegate Centre, Sheffield;

Wilfred Harrison, Director of the Octagon Theatre, Bolton, for the Margaret Greg Centre shows for handicapped children in the community. Thanks also to Glyn Putwain and his management of these shows;

Barrie and Joan Stephenson; Barbara Gillie and the entire Harrogate Christian Fellowship for practical help towards enabling me to function as a puppeteer and produce this book (especially the children); Christine Chidgey; and my parents. The Puppet Centre Trust, Sue Martin and Penny Francis; Rosie Hawley and the Harrogate Gateway Club;

and to all others who have asked to see me perform, bought puppets and kept me in touch with their progress.

Acknowledgment is also made to:

New English Library for permission to quote from *Music and Imagination* by Aaron Copland; Victor Gollancz for permission to quote from *Therapy in Music for Handicapped Children* by Paul Nordoff and Clive Robbins; Hutchinson for

ACKNOWLEDGMENTS

permission to quote from *The Ghost in the Machine* by Arthur Koestler, reprinted by permission of A.D. Peters & Co. Ltd; And to the following for permission to use photographs: Ken Dawson; *The Yorkshire Evening Post;* Tim Evanson; Frank Newbould; Hartmut Topf; Gisa Fisher.

Introduction

The Puppeteer
Some questions about creativity and communication
Everyone a potentiality bank
Decision making
Identifying with the puppet
Assessment checklist
Artistic conviction
Conclusions

Introduction

Whether as parents or as practising specialists, we are all aware
that a great deal of progress is being made in the treatment of
mentally handicapped people, and we probably concentrate
our attention on the most obvious contributions made in the
educational or medical fields. We would not be foolish to
welcome also the contribution of the professional in the so-
called fine arts — I mean drawing, painting or ceramics — or the
crafts, although seeing it as a contribution of a somewhat
different kind. But what I am concerned with in this book is yet
another dimension. It is neither simply "art" nor simply
"education", but a whole experience. It is theatre, and a
special kind of theatre, that of the puppeteer.

The Puppeteer
The puppeteer is someone who makes his or her ideas concrete,
translating them from the drawing board into two or three
dimensions, which in turn must be brought to life in action as
the animated symbols we call puppets. These puppets find
meaning only in theatre, where they are sustained by the
creative energy of an artist who has something to say or do
which cannot come to anything unless brought into being in a
work made by her own hands. Performed in a mixture of
sounds, silences, images, suggestions of the unseen and the
seen, the whole is recognised, processed and organised by the
audience into the language of puppetry. We shall examine this
artifact the puppet, see it is a real thing to be touched and
handled; and observe the puppeteer as a living person, and the
audience as actual people who have chosen to work together to
create the sharing experience of theatre.

This book is essentially practical, following the passage of
ideas from their creative roots to their expression in

performance, as the result of decisions made by a professional puppeteer, and by mentally handicapped artists and audiences.

This book, then, is about sharing creative experience. But how does this apply to people who are mentally handicapped?

Some questions about creativity and communication

Are some people creative and others not? Is creativity a fact of life, an unassailable part of human existence or is it only a fashionable idea? If it *is* an essential part of human existence, are people who are mentally handicapped, or even severely mentally handicapped, creative too?

I start out with the conviction that *life is what happens when you are being creative*. One act stimulates the next. We all have a desire to make evident our feelings about life: not only those deepest feelings which make all life seem like high drama, but also those everyday feelings that need expressing too. Small responses lead to greater intimacy, a tentative utterance produces eagerness to communicate.

Put like that, the twin ideas of creativity and communication seem inseparable, which is interesting. Does the first pre-suppose the second? Does communication provide the motive for creation? It would certainly seem nonsensical to absorb all creativity into the development of an inner language, or to make all those props and puppets for oneself alone. Whatever the process, it is a fact that the puppeteer speaks out and tells others through the puppet what has been going on in her life, on the drawing board, in the workroom. Not every puppeteer is a deep thinker, but every puppeteer thinks and says and does. In fact she never stops thinking and saying and doing and the puppetry you see is evidence of it.

But does everyone think? Does everyone have ideas? Does everyone *do*? Does a mentally handicapped person do these things?

The point is that our expectations of mentally handicapped people are sometimes very low, so we exclude them from experiences. In doing so, we deprive them of the extra care and stimulation they might need to spark off each precious creative impulse.

This book is about *having* expectations, about creating

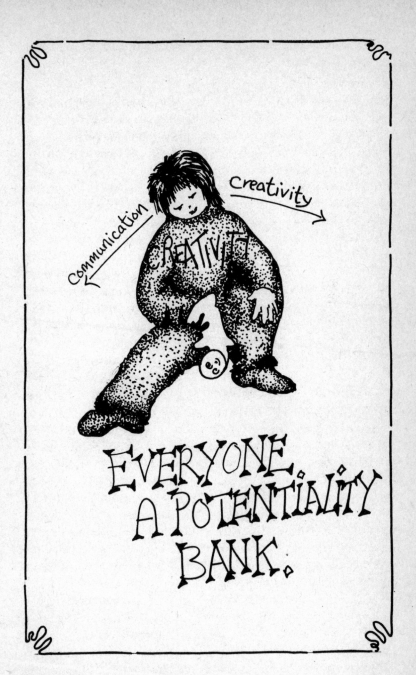

communication

creativity

EVERYONE
A POTENTIALITY
BANK.

expectations, and about the excitement of mutual response through puppetry.

Everyone a potentiality bank

Expect the most and you will get the best, *expect* nothing and you will get little. If you work on the premise that the mentally handicapped person is as much a potentiality bank as the so-called "normal" person, then much can be achieved. Much, much more. *Expect* a mentally handicapped person to have thoughts which can be expressed, because he is a creative being. But there are conditions. First, we must be prepared to look for this potential for communication; second, there must be people to hear, help and care for the person.

Stimulation must come from the very positive effect of having someone there who wants to listen (or watch) what you have to say when you choose to communicate. How many miserable people throw up ther hands in frustration and exclaim "What's the point—you never listen anyway!" Imagine a world in which no one ever listened to anyone else, or cared what was being said *ever*. In every walk of life we are dealing with human potential to create, to communicate and to form relationships. Without those expectations life itself becomes absurd and meaningless.

If an artist is going to make a contribution to the life of the person who is mentally handicapped, her attitudes have to be carefully thought out. It is not possible to work effectively as an artist in therapy if you hold a low view of life itself, or if you believe there is for some people "a life not worth living". As we shall see, puppetry is a healing activity as well as an educational one. If you believe that there *is* a life worth living and as a therapist or artist you are prepared to work to allow others to avail themselves of their own creativity, then you may respond to the view of Leonard Cohen, poet and song writer, who calls art "the only kind of expression that can heal"; or to that of Francis Bacon, Elizabethan philosopher, who wrote that "Man by the Fall fell at the same time from his state of innocence and from his dominion over nature. Both of these losses, however, can even in this life be in some part repaired; the former by religion and faith, the latter by the arts and sciences"; or to that of Aaron Copland, composer, who believes that "You cannot make art out of fear and suspicion; you can make it only out of affirmative beliefs. This sense of affirmation can be had only in part from one's inner being; for the rest it must be continually reactivated by a creative and yea-saying atmosphere in the life about one. The artist [*able or handicapped*] should feel himself affirmed and buoyed up by his community. In other words, art and the life of art must mean something, in the deepest sense, to the everyday citizen." (My parentheses C.A.B.)

If you can be trusted—as a puppeteer—to treat people as real human beings and therefore as precious, and expect them to affirm their humanity through art, then puppetry is one very important area of self-expression.

Puppeteers working in therapy must also recognise their responsibility as artists to strive for the highest professional standards, and to make rigorous attempts to lead the art of handicapped people out of the cottage industry era into the late twentieth century. Artists working in this area need to know about *this* community: about the media; the real issues of today; about drama and the theatre; about puppetry. Vital puppetry is neither a consolation nor a refuge, but, if it is used meaningfully, it will be distinguished by its relevance, by its power, and by its sheer appropriateness as a means for a mentally handicapped person to express himself.

Decision making

To treat the puppet as merely a visual aid—though it might be used as one under some circumstances—would be as mindless as playing a violin for arm exercises! Puppetry as a means to some other end other than self-expression limits the opportunity to express ideas. If we are going to treat the mentally handicapped person as a person with integrity, we have not only to be concerned with mechanical actions and craft techniques but with the thoughts behind the actions.

Although the puppeteer is engaged in many different activities, first of all to produce the puppet and then to perform with it, ultimately the reason for her work is to bring her into contact with others—to share. Without that objective there would be no sense to the preparation. The performance happens, grows out of the decisions made by different people in order to share the creative experience. (Note that the audience have a part in the performance too.) The thrill in performance, including in the advance preparation, involves as many different artistic choices as there are individuals. Without making decisions it is impossible to grow. Some people are not only prevented from maturing by the very nature of their handicap, but also through rarely having to make responsible decisions for themselves. Although every creative activity involves decision-making, puppetry is particularly useful therapeutically. In combining intrinsically so many art-forms, puppetry is at once flexible and sociable, offering great scope to people who may have a chance of developing expertise only in one very small area. Several people investing their different skills have to work together.

Making decisions creates tension and excitement, and a change from the bland experiences which make up the routine of many people who are handicapped. To cause something, to make something happen, these could be new experiences provided by presenting a performance—and these activities happen from both the audience and the performance angle. Passivity and contentment are often used as criteria for fulfilment. It is a trap. Achievement can come only through personal activity. Claiming lack of creativity as an excuse for inactivity is an excuse; creativity does not come in degrees but is a matter of fact—the ability to express oneself is where fresh opportunities and new experiences can shape latent skills.

The puppeteer's technique is at the most basic his mastery of puppets in their making and execution. However, these things are inseparable from his thought as a puppeteer. The real problems lie in the substance of what he is saying through the performance. It is not possible at this point to regard the puppeteer simply as a craftsman—he is *thinking* puppets, and expressing and creating human values. These values, although primarily concerned with the beauty and appropriateness of what he is saying and how he is saying it with the puppets, are still of deep psychological and human significance. This does not mean to say that what a person is saying is morally right—the artist, able or handicapped, is as likely to be "wrong" as anyone else. The important point is that teaching can lead a handicapped person to say things about his life and feelings through the medium of puppets, and not simply to make correct movements with them.

Identifying with the puppet

A mentally handicapped person can be hampered in his ability to relate to a puppet if the puppet is not effective—that is, with vividly designed features, particularly facial details. In the early stages it is helpful to present your group with finished characters, as it is not appropriate for many handicapped people to make their own puppets. The most severely handicapped people will not be able to identify with what they have made themselves—they tend to continue to see them as bits and pieces, unconnected components, not as a whole. "Let's pretend" is not necessarily something that comes naturally to a student, and although animation does not depend on the puppet having a visible face it does depend on the puppet having imagined human qualities. A figure with a face will encourage a person in what is expected of him. Essentially what you are doing is helping someone to say:

"The puppet is alive like me;
"He has a face, I have a face too;
"He moves, I move too";

Of course the puppet does not have to be a doll in order to have a face. The teacher can stick self-adhesive features on any object, and the statements above can remain true. If you do this, name the "characters", for example: "Mr Book", "This is Mr Wooden Spoon", "Here is Miss Mop".

The first task of the teacher is to develop the imaginative capacities of the students by simply encouraging them to recognise an object and to imagine it is alive, relating themselves and their bodies to the puppet, to lend their human qualities to the puppet.

Use the following statements:
"The puppet has eyes like me.
"Look, what has he seen?
"He can see like me
"He can move like me.

"Where is he going?

"He can jump like me.

"How high can he jump?

"Up to the ceiling."

However it is difficult to relate to bodily features or functions of others if your image of your own body is ill-defined or confused. To develop physical and psychological self-awareness, you may have to begin with more specific exercises identifying parts of the puppet's body and matching them with parts of the student's body. Encourage the students to look, to touch, and perhaps to talk about it.

Gradually you will be able to develop use of the puppet in drama. Many mentally handicapped people are unable to sustain imaginative play in ordinary drama because they lose concentration very quickly. The use of props and costume can reinforce the activity by "reminding" a person of what he is doing, but sometimes this is not adequate. Some people are unable to put *themselves* into an imaginary situation, especially if their image of themselves is at all fragmented and insecure. For them the puppet, because it is something outside themselves, a bundle of rags on a stick, may be liberating; here, a good face on the puppet helps the student to understand that just as he himself can do things in real life, so this little puppet character can too. The student begins to learn that he has control of this puppet, is master of the puppet, and through his control he can give it life. Unlike the situation in ordinary drama when the "actor" is "being someone", and is thus left vulnerable and unprotected, the puppet is an object, and can help the student to attain enough protective distance to express himself.

However, merely to present the student with good, lively puppets, and to get them relating happily to them, is not enough. A great deal of care needs still to go into the preparation for, and structuring of, a session and this is illustrated by the following story from my own experience.

Toothache:

This was a project designed to introduce puppetry to a club for mentally handicapped people. We started by telling the club members a story:

> Gregory was a green dragon. He was cared for by his Granny who was also a dentist. Gregory had to remember to clean his teeth. One day he chased Hilary the Witch and made her cross. She took her revenge by sending the Sugar and Spice Ladies . . . Gregory snapped them up one at a time and he was so full that he went to sleep without cleaning his teeth. During the night horrible bacteria invaded Gregory's mouth—nibbling and gnawing at his teeth—and in the morning he had TOOTHACHE! Granny took a look and with her special toothbrush she chased away the bacteria. Gregory always remembered to clean his teeth after that!

The story is very simple, and you will see from the drawings that the puppets too were very simply constructed. These were to be created out of kits which I had packed up. Each kit contained exactly what was needed for each puppet—tools as well as materials. So we distributed the kits, and showed how they were to be used. Some of the club members enjoyed putting the puppets together, as the materials were varied and unusual.

But many of the students found themselves unable to identify with the characters they were making. They could not see that they were making a character—it was just sequins, and a sock. Put together, they made in *my* mind a bacteria puppet, but to the club members who were mentally handicapped they remained meaningless.

As a consequence, some of the parents literally took over the making of the puppets, so that the members themselves simply wandered away, probably bored.

Then came the actual performance. It was clear that many members did not understand the story, or what they were doing holding the puppets at all. This put the final seal on disaster. Young women holding up the Sugar and Spice Ladies had to be steered into position, with their handbag in one hand and the puppet in the other; Gregory the Dragon was carried on stage and stood until someone else pulled him off or pushed him somewhere else. If instructions were shouted loudly enough some activity ensued, but the correct antics at the right moment were not all that was required. No one got the essence

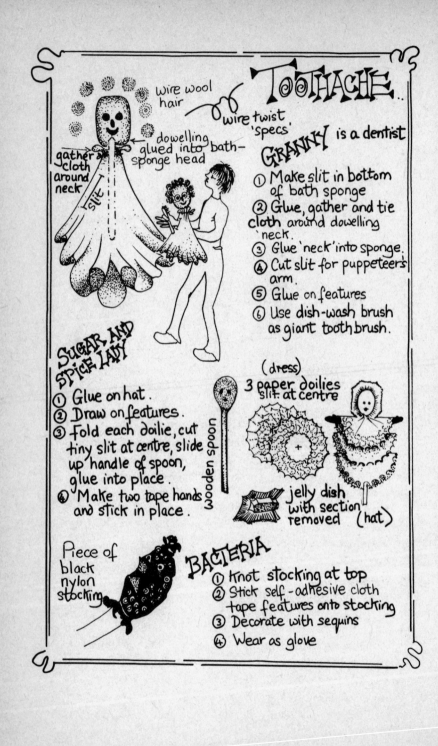

TOOTHACHE

wire wool hair

wire twist 'specs'

dowelling glued into bath-sponge head

gather cloth around neck

slit

GRANNY is a dentist

① Make slit in bottom of bath sponge
② Glue, gather and tie cloth around dowelling 'neck'
③ Glue 'neck' into sponge.
④ Cut slit for puppeteer's arm.
⑤ Glue on features
⑥ Use dish-wash brush as giant tooth brush.

SUGAR AND SPICE LADY

① Glue on hat.
② Draw on features.
③ Fold each doilie, cut tiny slit at centre, slide up handle of spoon, glue into place.
④ Make two tape hands and stick in place.

wooden spoon

(dress)
3 paper doilies slit at centre

jelly dish with section removed (hat)

BACTERIA

Piece of black nylon stocking

① Knot stocking at top
② Stick self-adhesive cloth tape features onto stocking
③ Decorate with sequins
④ Wear as glove

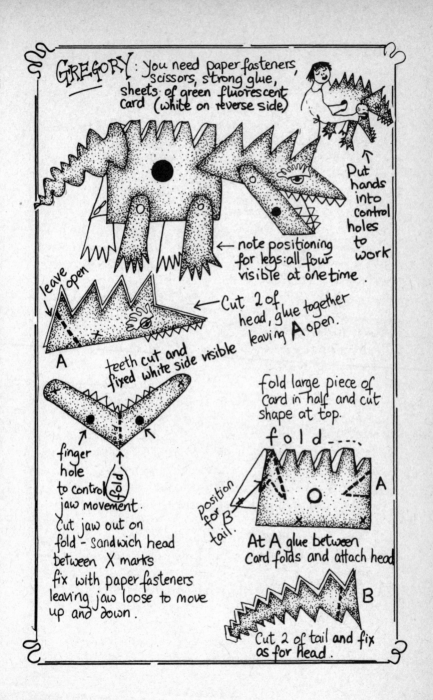

GREGORY: You need paper fasteners, scissors, strong glue, sheets of green fluorescent card (white on reverse side)

Put hands into control holes to work

← note positioning for legs: all four visible at one time.

leave open

← Cut 2 of head, glue together leaving A open.

A

teeth cut and fixed white side visible

finger hole to control jaw movement.

fold

Cut jaw out on fold – sandwich head between X marks fix with paper fasteners leaving jaw loose to move up and down.

fold large piece of card in half and cut shape at top.

f o l d - - - - -

A

position for B tail.

At A glue between card folds and attach head

B

Cut 2 of tail and fix as for head.

of the exercise—that is, that puppets are a means through which the person *speaks*.

What do we mean when we talk about wanting a person to speak through the puppets?

What we are talking about here is an aesthetic judgment. It is comparatively easy to make a judgment on the basis of craftsmanship or manual dexterity. But how does one make aesthetic judgments? The person who must make these judgments is the artist himself—step by step, by being critical at the moment of creation. A creative act is a self-critical act. If our objective is to encourage a mentally handicapped person in his creative thinking, then we need a checklist for ourselves with which to draw attention to the important points. What we are looking at is the *use* of the puppet. So we observe the manipulator with a puppet, and look for the following points:

Assessment Checklist
1. Relationship between puppet and puppeteer: is there a relationship, and how does it work?
2. The way the manipulator is prepared to fulfil his obligations to use the puppet to show to others (puppetry as a performing art): is he sharing the experience?
3. The way he rises to the expectations of others as they show the desire to see him play (social relationship with the audience). How is he communicating with others?
4. The use of the puppet to extend his social repertoire: communication, intellectual content, expression of feelings, making moral choices.
5. The appropriateness of his actions with the puppet (dramatic consistence of his presentation of the puppet character).
6. Sensitivity to the situation (to the current audience response).

By all these criteria the experience of "Toothache" was a dismal failure. Not only had we failed to create the circumstances for the students to act for themselves, they had actually had the initiative taken out of their hands. And to interfere with a person's own capacity to act is to deny him his dignity . . .

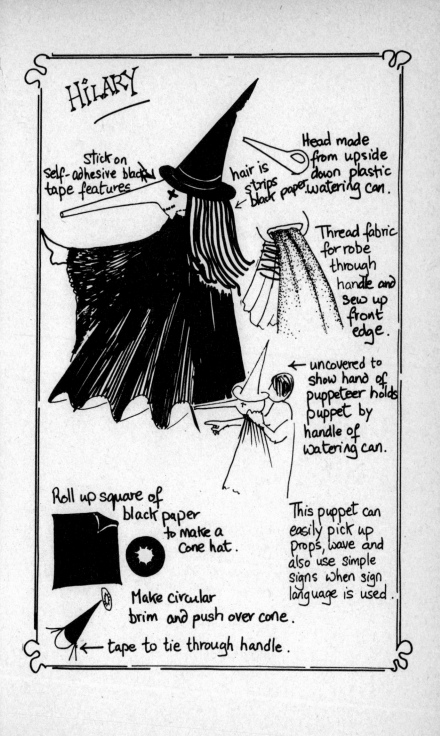

HILARY

Stick on self-adhesive black tape features

hair is strips black paper

Head made from upside down plastic watering can.

Thread fabric for robe through handle and sew up front edge.

← uncovered to show hand of puppeteer holds puppet by handle of watering can.

Roll up square of black paper to make a cone hat.

This puppet can easily pick up props, wave and also use simple signs when sign language is used.

Make circular brim and push over cone.

← tape to tie through handle.

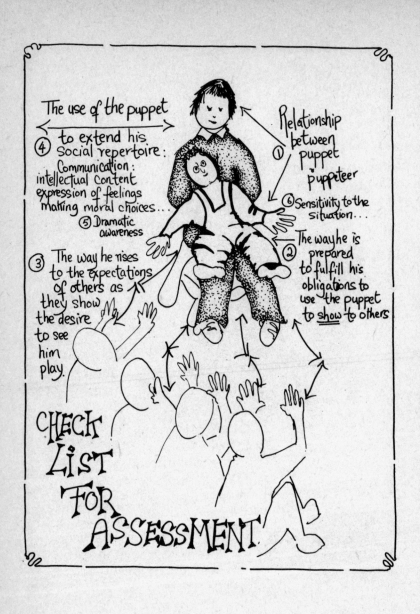

The use of the puppet
to extend his social repertoire:
④ Communication:
intellectual content
expression of feelings
making moral choices...
⑤ Dramatic awareness

① Relationship between puppet & puppeteer

⑥ Sensitivity to the situation...

② The way he is prepared to fulfill his obligations to use the puppet to show to others

③ The way he rises to the expectations of others as they show the desire to see him play.

CHECK LIST FOR ASSESSMENT

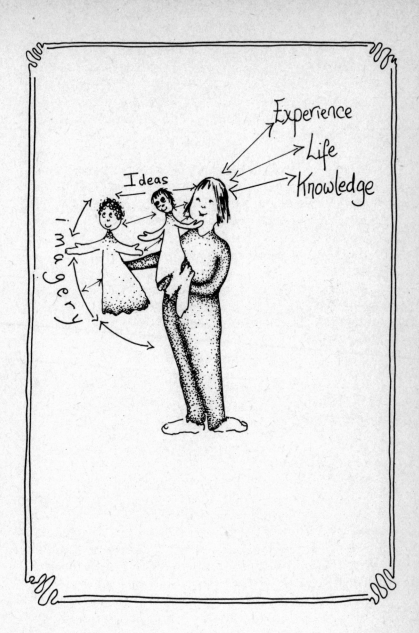

Experience

Life

Knowledge

Ideas

imagery

It is therefore important to plan the sessions step by step, working from where each person is in his personal development according to the checklist.

In concrete terms, from the experience with "Toothache" I learned that before ever I started I should have asked myself the following questions:

1. First of all, what do the group on the project know about teeth and their care? What do they know about the effect of sugar on teeth, or about bacteria? Before anyone can express ideas they have to have some grasp of the relevant information.

2. Having understood the facts, then the facts have to be related to the imagery in the story, that is to the puppets. Is it understood that the bacteria in the information about teeth care are being represented by puppets? Is it clear that the Sugar and Spice Ladies represent the sugar in the information?

3. Are teeth cleaning, toothache, and visits to the dentist within the experience of each group member?

Ideas grow out of knowledge and experience. If these elements are missing, then ideas will not be expressed.

Artistic conviction

Creative expression gives coherence—personal coherence to the individual, even when her relationship to the outside world may be confused or apparently irrelevant. Artistic expression particularises who we are as individuals. By using language in a variety of ways—movement as well as speech—we present our ideas and convictions to others and form relationships. Whatever language we use—puppets or some other art-form —artistic expression makes experience concrete and available for others to receive. It gives us the coherence we need to be understood by others, but also to know ourselves better. So there cannot be true artistic expression without conviction.

A manager of a training centre once asked me whether puppetry could be used to teach sex education to the trainees. I concluded that it would not work because in that centre sexuality was something no one ever talked openly about. The trainees had no convictions at all on the subject. They were never encouraged to ask questions or discuss their feelings. Their sexuality existed only as animal behaviour in the eyes of those responsible for their education. It existed outside the framework of human *relationships*.

Can we really encourage people who are mentally handicapped to have firm convictions and to hold to positive philosophies, such as Aaron Copland sees as essential to artistic expression? This is indeed an ideal for which to aim, so be prepared to affirm each person in what he thinks and does in art, by being supportive and caring. Our aim should not be just to *do puppetry*, but to work *with puppeteers* who are mentally handicapped.

Conclusions

As a performing artist, then, one can never never look at the puppet alone, nor at the performer alone, nor at the audience alone. Puppetry is a performance art and so contains all the variety of opportunities for participation by anyone. The common ground on which we all stand is that we all have potential to communicate, and to involve ourselves in our own creative capacity—some needing more help than others. Confidence in this potential gives me as a performing artist who has chosen to work with people who are handicapped the optimism to persist even with those whose response is slow, in anticipation of a response growing secretly within the student. Belief in this potential is vital to the work, but so is an uncluttered view of puppetry as a performance art.

One might say that exhibition art is for things shown while performance art is for actions shown. In exhibition art the artistic activity ends with the completion and showing of the object. Puppetry as a performance art only starts when the puppet is complete—which unfortunately is the point where most people finish!

A major aim of this book must be to dispel the fears most people have about performing with puppets, and to give teachers, therapists and parents clear guidance on how to use puppets as a means of artistic expression. Handicap of any kind inevitably means separation from the self in terms of self-awareness, and separation from the rest of society too. The reality of creativity is reconciliation: the harmonising of personalities and conditions which at first glance would seem incompatible. A performing art, puppetry does to an extent realise capacities to share and form relationships through art, and to this extent it is a healing activity.

PART ONE

The Puppet

Exercises in animation
Making your first puppets
The glove puppet
The rod puppet
The dual control puppet
Use the ancient puppet traditions
  Types of marionette
  Shadow puppets
  Bunraku puppets
Shadow puppetry via the over-head projector
Going on to the big shadow screen
A note on junk puppetry

The Puppet

WELL, what is a puppet? What happens to a puppet to make it come alive? Let us forget for a moment about traditional puppets—dolls—because the universal attraction of puppets does not depend on the puppet being as like an animal or human being as possible. We are now talking about *animation* and not just *puppetry*. If you look up these two words in the dictionary you will find that the definitions are very different. And most of us would have no difficulty in deciding which is more attractive.

animate—to give life to; to enliven; to enspirit; to actuate.
animated—lively, full of spirit: moving as if alive.
puppetry—play of or with puppets; anything like or associated with puppets.

Exercises in animation—helping ideas to grow
You will need:
An overhead projector
pairs of scissors
knife
fork
a tangle of string

On pages 34 and 35 are storyboards for you to follow. As you become more experienced you will be able to work spontaneously off the screen in front of your group, but until then prepare first by sketching out your own ideas scene by scene.

As you follow the instructions with each picture you will be giving life to inanimate objects—making them move as if alive.

We have already begun to animate objects in the section "Identifying with the puppet", but here are some more ideas.

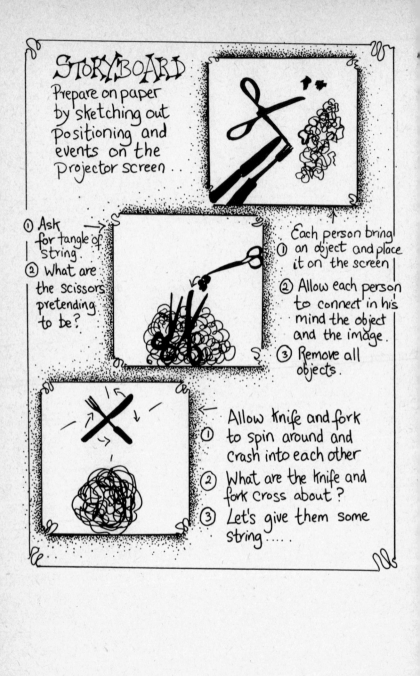

STORYBOARD

Prepare on paper by sketching out positioning and events on the projector screen..

① Ask for tangle of string.
② What are the scissors pretending to be?

Each person bring
① an object and place it on the screen
② Allow each person to connect in his mind the object and the image.
③ Remove all objects.

Allow knife and fork
① to spin around and crash into each other
② What are the knife and fork cross about?
③ Let's give them some string....

STORYBOARD CONT.

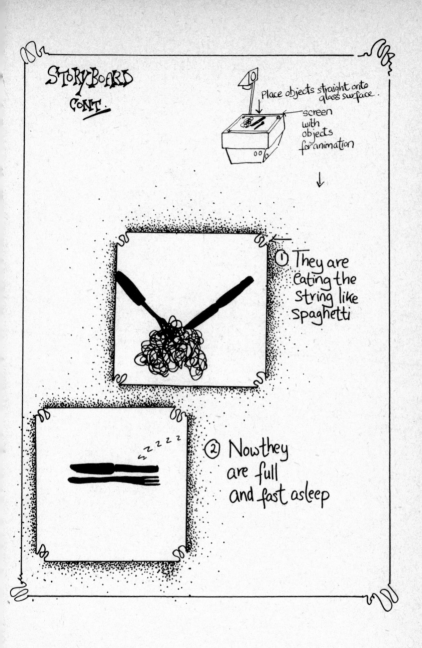

Place objects straight onto glass surface.

screen with objects for animation

① They are eating the string like spaghetti

② Now they are full and fast asleep

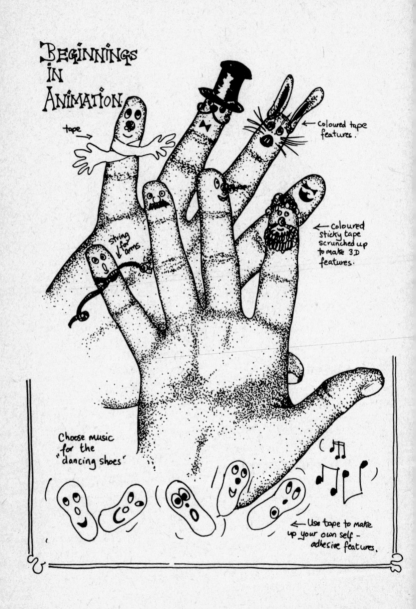

BEGINNINGS IN ANIMATION

tape →

← coloured tape features.

← coloured sticky tape scrunched up to make 3D features.

string for arms

Choose music for the "dancing shoes"

← Use tape to make up your own self-adhesive features.

Take off your shoes. Take them for "a walk" to "meet" each other.

Stick features on the shoes. Find anything else in the room that attracts you to use.

Chase around with things that have suddenly "come alive".

Draw features on your fingers. Wiggling decorated fingers to each other is especially good for people who may never have played with their fingers and toes as children.

This brings us on to another point, that of play. Play is important, but it is not the prime ingredient of puppetry. Animation is an imaginative activity, and play is not necessarily imaginative. But of course animation and play are intertwined in a most exciting way in puppetry. Our understanding of puppetry as an art is confused if we merely invite people to play with puppets. Some free play may take place, but that will not represent the art of puppetry. Puppetry is a performing art.

With the projector, in a single simple activity we moved from two, into three, into two dimensions and back again. We have refreshed our ideas on puppetry. True expression of our creativity takes us on a journey. We can take a handicapped person on this journey with us. Put away your stuffed toys, your television frogs and bears and come a new way!

Making your first puppets

There are already some fine books available about puppet-making, but you will need a slightly different approach if you work with mentally handicapped students. The puppets that follow are designed along certain guidelines developed to make puppetry readily available as a "language" to people whose skill in communication is impoverished by handicap.

We have already experimented using an overhead projector. For that experiment to work we had to follow the transformation of a three-dimensional object into two dimensions on the screen. For a person to work puppets he has to have that ability, he has to be able to follow the transference from one dimension into the other and back again: that is, he has to have a degree of symbolic understanding. Using the overhead

HEADS

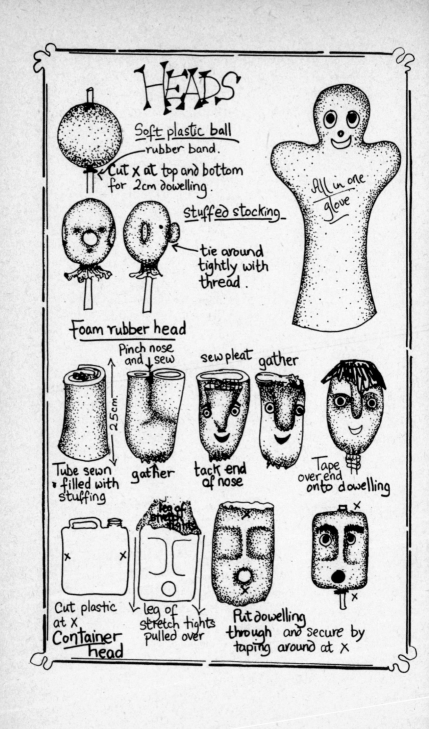

Soft plastic ball

rubber band.

Cut X at top and bottom for 2cm dowelling.

stuffed stocking

tie around tightly with thread.

All in one glove

Foam rubber head

Pinch nose and sew

sew pleat

gather

25 cm.

Tube sewn & filled with stuffing

gather

tack end of nose

Tape over end onto dowelling

Cut plastic at X

Container head

leg of tights

leg of stretch tights pulled over

Put dowelling through and secure by taping around at X

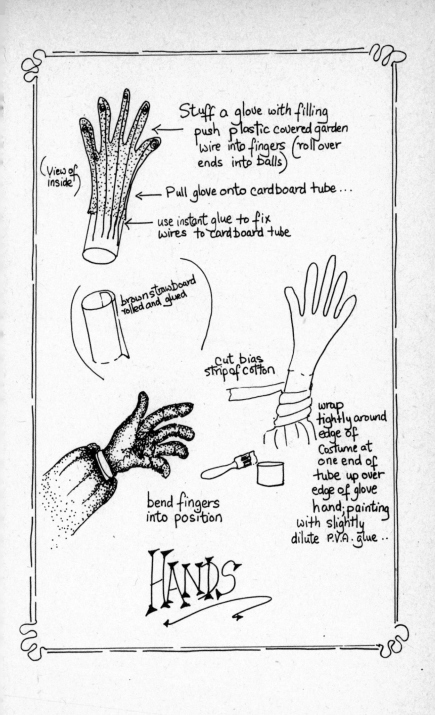

Stuff a glove with filling push plastic covered garden wire into fingers (roll over ends into balls)

(View of inside)

Pull glove onto cardboard tube...

use instant glue to fix wires to cardboard tube

brown strawboard rolled and glued

Cut bias strip of cotton

wrap tightly around edge of costume at one end of tube up over edge of glove hand; painting with slightly dilute P.V.A. glue ..

bend fingers into position

HANDS

HANDS cont...

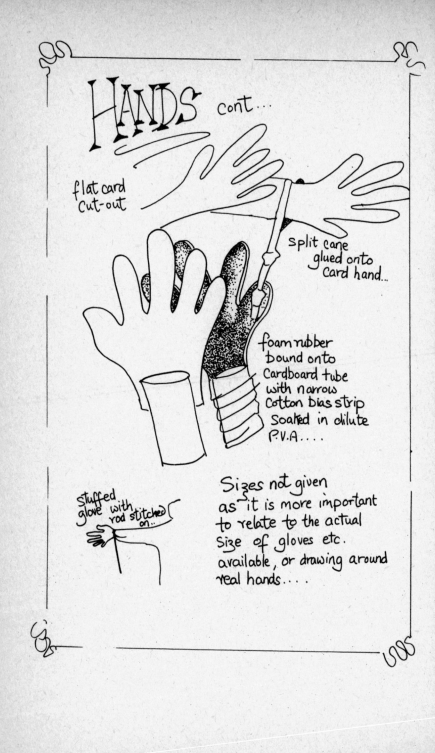

flat card
cut-out

split cane
glued onto
card hand...

foam rubber
bound onto
Cardboard tube
with narrow
Cotton bias strip
Soaked in dilute
P.V.A....

Stuffed
glove with
rod stitched
on...

Sizes not given
as it is more important
to relate to the actual
Size of gloves etc.
available, or drawing around
real hands....

NOSES

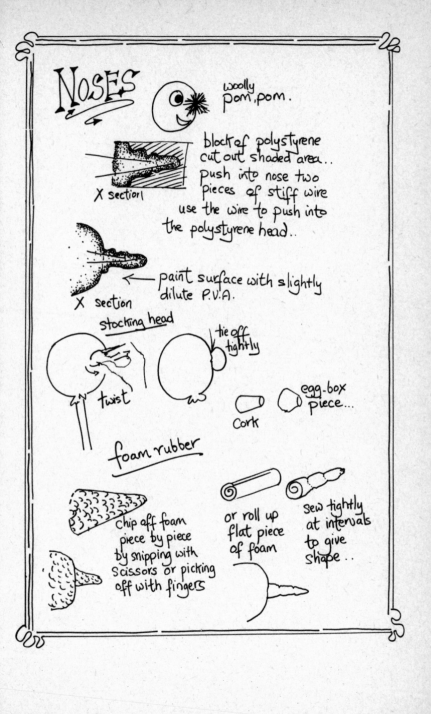

woolly pom, pom.

block of polystyrene
cut out shaded area..
push into nose two
pieces of stiff wire
use the wire to push into
the polystyrene head..

X section

X section

← paint surface with slightly dilute P.V.A.

stocking head

twist

tie off tightly

Cork

egg-box piece...

foam rubber

Chip off foam piece by piece by snipping with scissors or picking off with fingers

or roll up flat piece of foam

sew tightly at intervals to give shape..

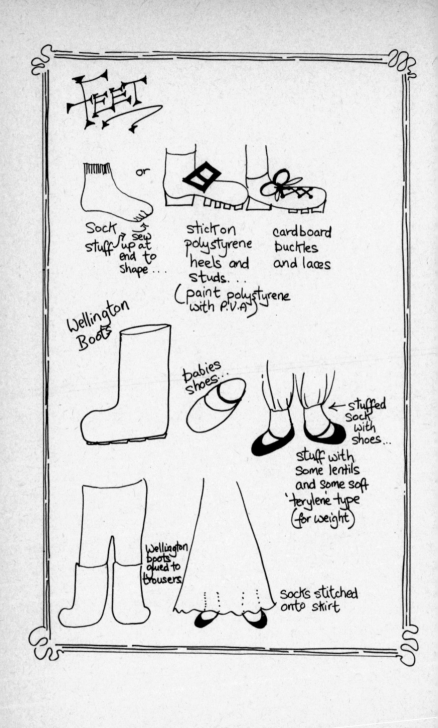

FEET

Sock stuff, sew up at end to shape...

or

stick on polystyrene heels and studs...
(paint polystyrene with P.V.A.)

cardboard buckles and laces

Wellington Boots

babies shoes...

← stuffed sock with shoes...

stuff with some lentils and some soft 'terylene' type (for weight)

Wellington boots glued to trousers

socks stitched onto skirt

EXPRESSION

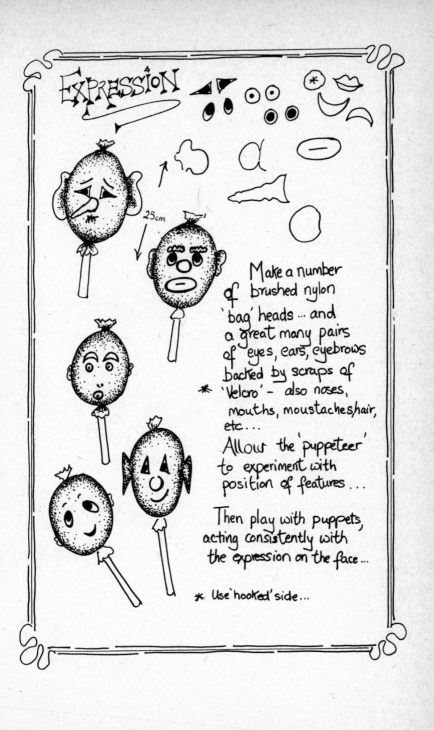

Make a number of brushed nylon 'bag' heads ... and a great many pairs of eyes, ears, eyebrows backed by scraps of 'Velcro' * - also noses, mouths, moustaches, hair, etc...

Allow the 'puppeteer' to experiment with position of features...

Then play with puppets, acting consistently with the expression on the face...

* Use 'hooked' side...

.25cm.

projector can help him to do that. When he is able to follow the story, then to take part himself and spontaneously to bring objects to place on the screen, he is ready to go on to the next stage.

Guidelines (pages 38–43)

First, make your collection of things to work with:

Collect suitable old clothing;

Make up collections of hands and feet (Simply collect gloves of different kinds and also socks and shoes);

Collect the heads from old toys or make your own;

Make up a collection of facial features and keep them all separate: noses, eyes, mouths, eyebrows, ears.

The most adaptable head is one that is fixed on a piece of dowelling—18mm (¾″) is the easiest to hold.

Also illustrated is the simple glove puppet (page 38).

However, I am careful about how I use glove puppets early on. Some glove puppets are unattractive when out of use. If they are very floppy and have no support other than the hand inside, the "collapse" when out of use offers little encouragement to pick it up again. It is important, if you are working with people who are not highly motivated, that the puppets are interesting and stimulating even when at rest. As a general guide, make your puppets colourful and characterful—and look for other ideas than the traditional glove puppet only.

Whenever possible, work with large puppets. The designs in this book have been developed over a number of years, with mentally handicapped people of all ages and abilities, and on the whole the larger sized puppets have proved to be the most successful. One reason for this is that they provide a greater challenge to the user. It seems to be easier to relate to a larger puppet. It can be incorporated into ordinary activities—children invite the puppet to tea, put nappies on the puppet and "change" him, the puppet can "play" with toys with a child, he may even "draw" pictures; and older people enjoy mothering the puppet as if it were a young child.

The point cannot be made emphatically enough that puppetry is a performing art. So the first problems in puppetry to be considered are:

The group performing and the group being performed to.

This means that any discussion about puppet-making is relevant only in order to facilitate either of the above. Puppet-making should not be seen as an opportunity to make things—this is another kind of activity. The object in puppetry has to be *performance*.

Most of these puppets are thus made in advance by the teacher or therapist. However, in many instances it is a good idea to have detachable features, or half completed puppets, and then as part of an initial game to put the puppet together. Experiment with the positions of features to create different expressions. Features should be strongly made and kept together in categories. Use ways of fixing that do not require sewing or glue, unless the puppet is to be permanent: "Velcro", press-studs, double-sided carpet tape.

It is important not to depend on using puppets made by the people who are mentally handicapped. Some of these may be excellent, but, as my experience with the "Toothache" show demonstrates, the more severely handicapped people simply do not relate to their "home-made" puppets. Making a puppet does not automatically mean that it becomes meaningful, in fact in this case the reverse was true: the fact that the puppet began as separate components *prevented* identification with the character. Many ideas had gone into the actualisation of the ultimate puppet, but the thought processes had not originated with the person making the puppet. The puppets were very clearly designed, but the effort required to relate to the design of someone else and then to assimilate the character and events was too great.

The most successful puppets I have used have been professional ones, large, well designed and often already seen in a show, or in the hands of a skilled person.

Here are two essential principles to help you to design and make effective puppets:

1. Just as a poet expresses his thoughts using word imagery, so the puppeteer uses puppet imagery. The puppets express something of the puppeteer.
2. The look of the puppet reinforces the character of the puppet.

Here are some character sketches for a show, "Boris the Bad", which has been performed in hospitals, hospital schools, ESN(M) and (S) schools as well as for children in ordinary schools and university students.

King—loud, greedy:	brightly coloured richly textured clothes. White wig, bright, big yellow boots. Fat.
Peter—foolish, lovable, affectionate;	rustic colours, uncoordinated, leggings, mass of untidy hair, big foolish mouth.
Fag End Lil, mother of King— busy, always sweeping up:	white hair in bun, quite thin, patchwork costume, cigarette in mouth, permanently attached to up sweeping brush.

When you make a puppet, therefore, hunt out fabric for its character value for the character you are building. Each character should be an individual, and so choose costume and features as you might choose clothes and accessories for yourself.

Whether the puppet is to be used in a "show" or to be seen with the puppeteer at the "front", the character of the puppet must be effective enough to make the relationship between puppeteer and puppet convincing. Inconsistency between the puppet and his appearance makes a performance superficial.

Features

Features in professional puppets are very clear. They should be pronounced, yet not seem stereotyped. Once again you should consider the character. Mouths do not have to articulate, but they can still have a shape to suit the character of the puppet.

Although any object can be animated and be brought "to life" to take part in some fantasy of our imagination, the puppet is an object designed especially to be animated. It is designed to "become" a certain character, and to perform certain actions. Scope must be given to the puppet *to act*.

The glove puppet (page 47)

Can pick up objects, move them around, clap hands, hit, embrace.

SIMPLE GLOVE PUPPETS.

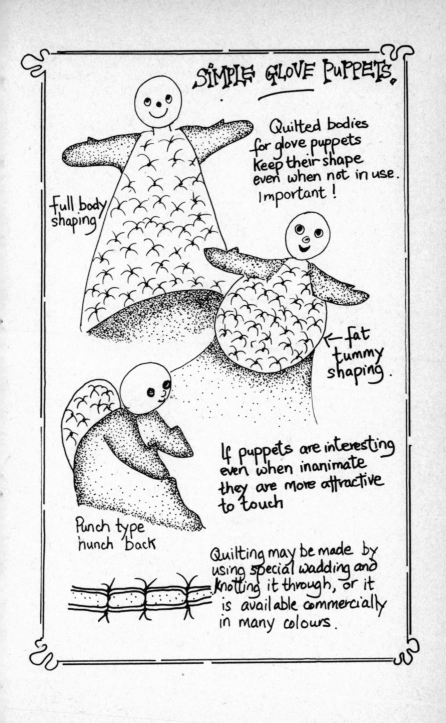

Quilted bodies
for glove puppets
keep their shape
even when not in use.
Important!

Full body
shaping

←fat
tummy
shaping.

If puppets are interesting
even when inanimate
they are more attractive
to touch

Punch type
hunch back

Quilting may be made by
using special wadding and
knotting it through, or it
is available commercially
in many colours.

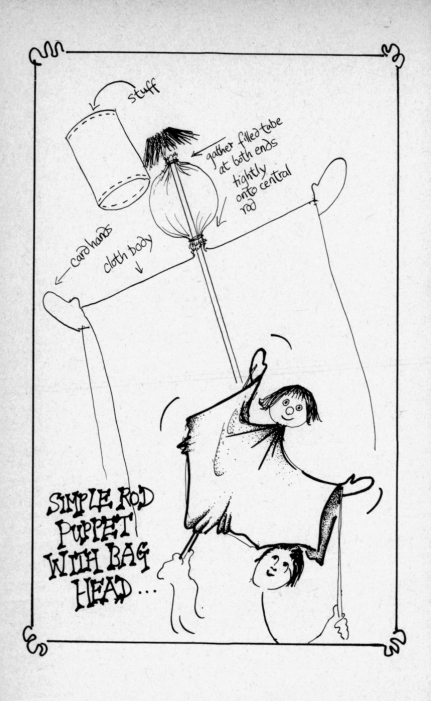

stuff

gather filled tube at both ends tightly onto central rod

← card hands

cloth body ↓

SIMPLE ROD PUPPET WITH BAG HEAD ...

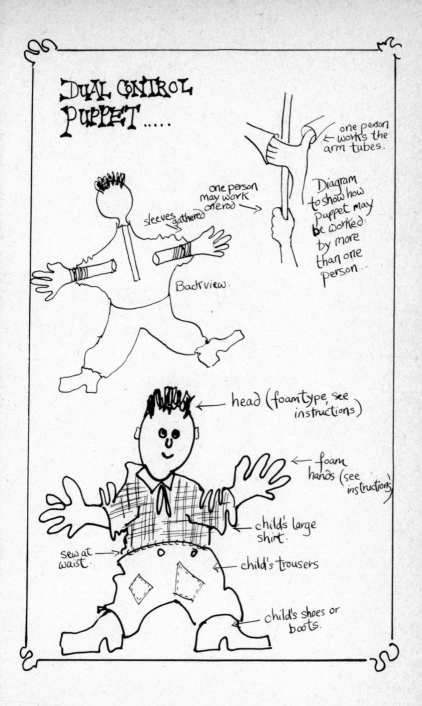

DUAL CONTROL PUPPET .....

one person works the arm tubes.

Diagram to show how Puppet may be worked by more than one person...

one person may work one rod →

sleeves gathered

Back view.

head (foam type, see instructions)

foam hands (see instructions)

child's large shirt.

sew at waist.

child's trousers

child's shoes or boots.

MAKE A GIANT ROD PUPPET !

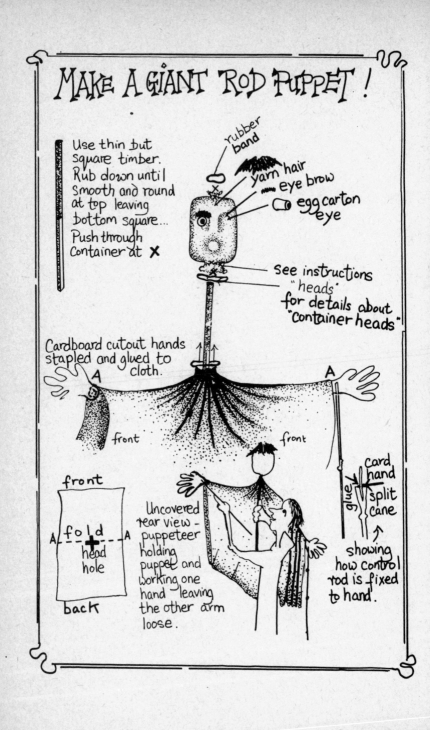

Use thin but square timber. Rub down until smooth and round at top leaving bottom square...
Push through Container at **X**

rubber band

yarn hair

eye brow

egg carton eye

see instructions "heads" for details about "container heads"

Cardboard cutout hands stapled and glued to cloth.

A

A

front

front

card hand

glue

split cane

showing how control rod is fixed to hand.

front

A — fold — A

head hole

back

Uncovered rear view - puppeteer holding puppet and working one hand leaving the other arm loose.

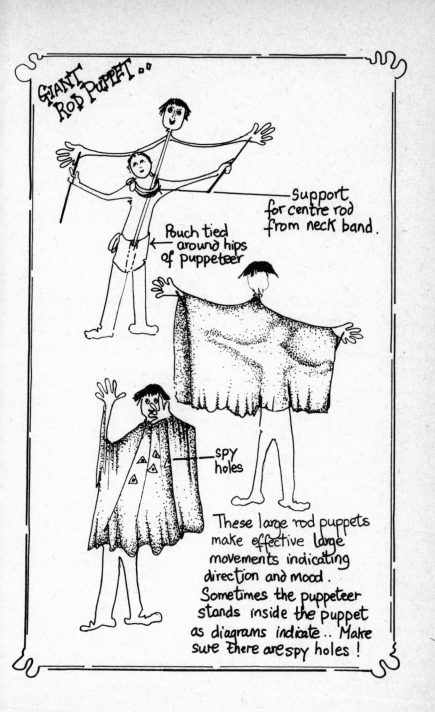

GIANT ROD PUPPET..

Support for centre rod from neck band.

Pouch tied around hips of puppeteer

spy holes

These large rod puppets make effective large movements indicating direction and mood. Sometimes the puppeteer stands inside the puppet as diagrams indicate.. Make sure there are spy holes!

The rod puppet (pages 48, 50, 51)

Is effective for making grand gestures, for dancing, whirling around, waving arms, pointing, but cannot very easily pick things up.

The dual-control puppet (page 49)

The dual-control, hand-rod puppet may be worked in close quarters with a handicapped person. It can pick things up, and do most of the things that an ordinary glove puppet can do, except that it is usually larger and is worked by two hands and effectively by two people. If one person works the puppet alone, and for the first time, he will probably be able only to jig the puppet around with the head rod, so it is important that the puppet looks convincing however he is worked.

Whatever type of puppet you make, choose a good cloth that is not too heavy but has stiffness, so that it retains enough shape to keep the puppet looking interesting even when not in motion. A good example is the plastic bottle puppet. This is a very tall puppet designed to be worn by the puppeteer on a body carrying band and a pectoral band (pages 50–51).

The body of the puppet can be made in any material—sometimes the structure is the costume, at other times the structure may be covered by the costume.

Try basket-work costume/structures, or knitted costumes, with double thickness rug wool on very large needles. It might be hard on the fingers, but it is effective!

In shorter puppets, quilting wadding or commercial quilting is ideal for adding to the body.

As you design and make your costumes, try to develop an eye for what is dramatic, and try to create effects. What do all the puppets look like together? Do they look good as a group? Many home-made puppets look insipid because the maker has forgotten to design individual characters to be seen at a *distance*: mould faces and costumes boldly and do not be afraid of over-exaggeration or caricature.

Look around at fabrics, contrast brocades with corduroy, denim with satin, velvets with lawns, georgettes and woollens, and keep the look of the costumes in mind as you plan the puppets. Look out for those extra trimmings: ribbon, lace, feathers, down.

A Rajasthani Marionette

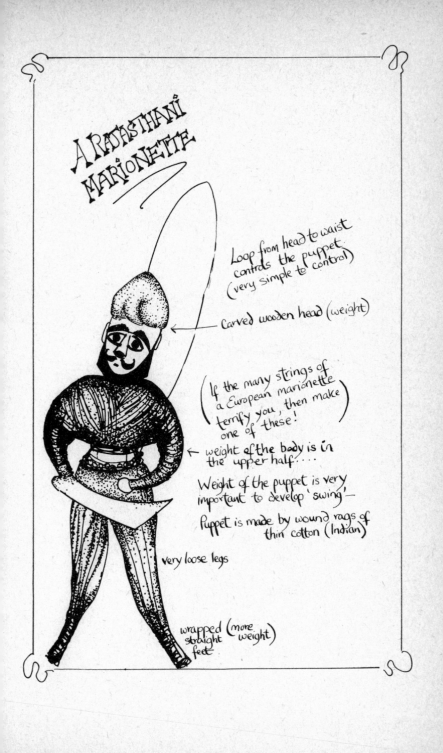

Loop from head to waist controls the puppet (very simple to control)

Carved wooden head (weight)

(If the many strings of a European marionette terrify you, then make one of these!)

weight of the body is in the upper half....

Weight of the puppet is very important to develop 'swing'

Puppet is made by wound rags of thin cotton (Indian)

very loose legs

wrapped straight feet (more weight)

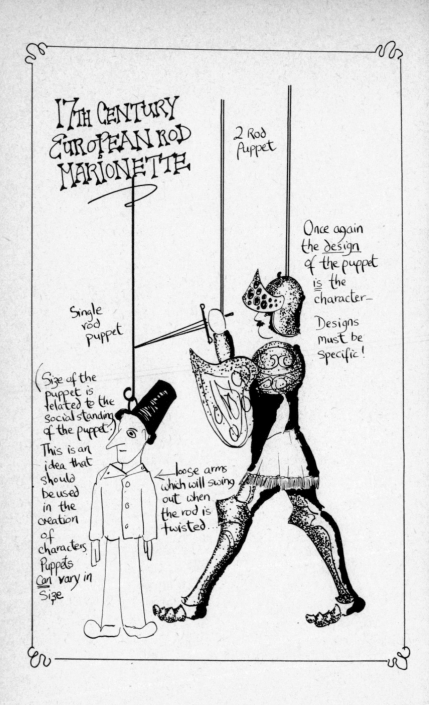

17TH CENTURY EUROPEAN ROD MARIONETTE

2 Rod Puppet

Single rod puppet

Once again the <u>design</u> of the puppet <u>is</u> the character —

Designs must be specific!

(Size of the puppet is related to the social standing of the puppet. This is an idea that should be used in the creation of characters. Puppets <u>can</u> vary in size

← loose arms which will swing out when the rod is twisted

The more colourful and exciting the puppets, the more stimulating they will be to the group you are leading. Are *you* excited about your puppet? That is an important question.

When you are preparing puppets for use with your group from the very start, see each as a character with his own individual characteristics. Each is a *real* personality—made up of typical materials that express that personality.

Use the ancient puppet traditions

It is always exciting to trace puppetry back into its historical past and to see how we can benefit now. To grasp some sense of the history of an art-form is a reminder that the psychology of art goes back thousands of years. In such a study we find first of all that human beings are *significant*: they have left signs of their activity and thought. What can we learn to help us to use puppets with people who are handicapped?

Types of marionette

Rajasthan in India is a place where some very simply manipulated marionettes are still used in performance today. They have carved wooden heads and bodies with stuffed rag-doll arms. The marionette is controlled by a single loop of string from the head to the waist and the arms are left free to swing about. Sometimes there is an extra loop attached to the hands for extra control. This design of marionette is simple in use—and yet the characters may be colourful and effective.

During the sixteenth and seventeenth centuries all over Europe were to be found marionettes suspended from a metal bar. This bar went right through the wooden body and was twisted to work the body—the arms were loose, as were the legs. The puppets varied in height according to their rank in society: a worker was about two feet high and a king about four feet! As an adaptation, other rods could be fixed to a hand or leg.

Shadow puppets

There is an interesting example of these in Java. The puppet-master, or *dalang*, as he is called, holds his puppets on perpen-

JAVANESE SHADOW PUPPET..

Note exaggerated size of shoulders — the important aspect of this puppet....

Whole puppet is rigid apart from arms... (no emphasis on the mouth as part of a functional head)

The expressiveness of the puppet rests in the arms.....

← joints (overlap)

Highly decorated, stylised human form.

← rod

rod →

Central rod

TURKISH SHADOW PUPPET

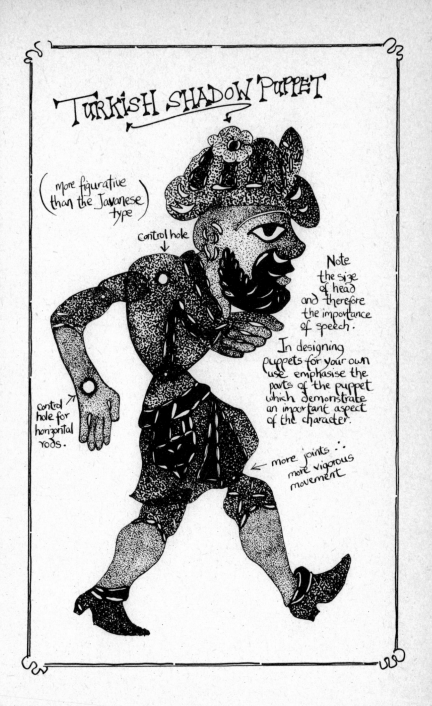

(more figurative than the Javanese type)

Control hole

Control hole for horizontal rods.

Note the size of head and therefore the importance of speech.

In designing puppets for your own use, emphasise the parts of the puppet which demonstrate an important aspect of the character.

more joints ∴ more vigorous movement

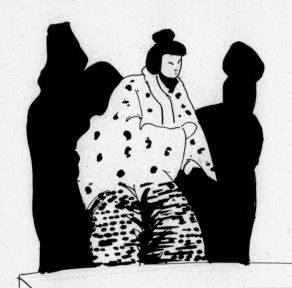

JAPANESE BUNRAKU PUPPET

One puppet
has more than one
operator — imagine in
your own situation how one
person's confidence and
ability to communicate could
be increased from working
with someone more experienced...

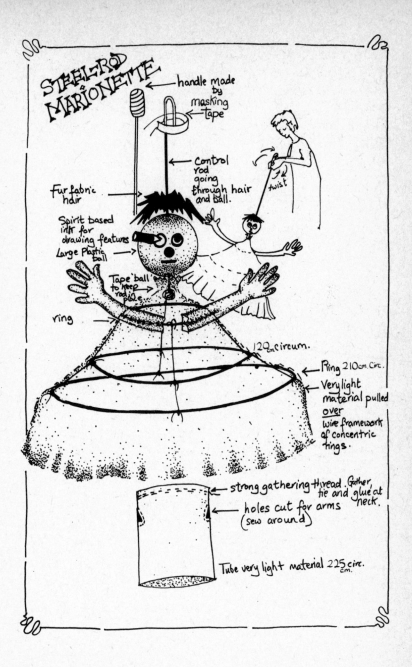

STEEL-ROD MARIONETTE

handle made by masking tape

control rod going through hair and ball.

twist

Fur fabric hair

Spirit based ink for drawing features

Large Plastic Ball

Tape 'ball' to keep rod in place.

ring

120 cm circum.

Ring 210cm. Circ.

Very light material pulled over wire framework of concentric rings.

strong gathering thread. Gather, tie and glue at neck.

holes cut for arms (sew around)

Tube very light material 225 circ. cm.

dicular bone rods against a white cotton screen. The shoulders of these puppets are very exaggerated and are depicted as a front view to show both arms hanging freely. The puppets are designed to be seen very clearly. These might appear to be highly stylised—but the emphasis is on the movement of the body.

As we move back towards the West, we find the puppets becoming more human and less animal-like, with the emphasis more on the spoken word. Heads tend to become larger and more exaggerated and the individuality of each puppet character more pronounced, as in the Turkish shadow puppet illustrated (page 57).

The Bunraku puppets of Japan

These puppets are interesting because one puppet is worked by at least three men. One person works the head, mouth, eyes and eyebrows and the right hand of the puppet. Another man works the left arm and hand, while another works the legs. The puppeteers are visible, though usually dressed in black. They are as much a part of the drama as the puppet. Their involvement is fascinating as you watch them acting and feeling for the puppets: if you imagine that the art of puppetry is simply that of waving a puppet around, the Bunraku puppeteers will convince you that it makes just as much demand on acting ability as does straight drama. These puppets are probably too complicated to work with people who are mentally handicapped, but the principle of having more than one manipulator is one that could be useful. Also, to have the manipulators on show can enable a person to understand that she is being seen, that her job is important. When we work with large puppets, a great deal of space is needed and the limits of the stage or booth are obvious, so we can make use of the fact that it is not necessary to conceal the puppeteer. The Bunraku theatre also uses a narrator and a musician. All aspects of the drama work in balance: narrator, puppets, puppeteer, musician are equally important. These too are ideas we can apply with mentally handicapped puppeteers.

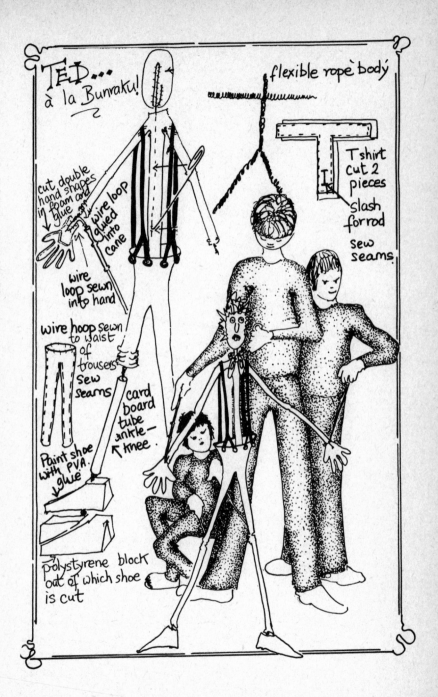

TED...
à la Bunraku!

flexible rope body

cut double hand shapes in foam card glue

wire loop glued into cane

wire loop sewn into hand

wire hoop sewn to waist of trousers

Sew seams

card board tube ankle→ knee.

Paint shoe with PVA. glue

polystyrene block out of which shoe is cut

Tshirt cut 2 pieces

slash for rod

sew seams.

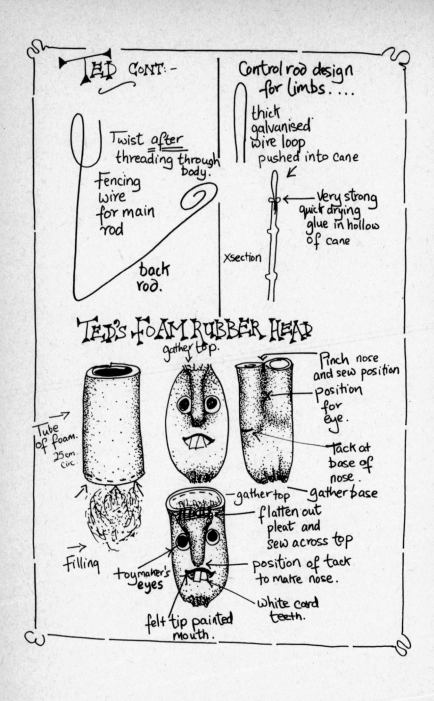

TED CONT:-

Twist **after** threading through body.

Fencing wire for main rod

back rod.

Control rod design for limbs. . . .

thick galvanised wire loop pushed into cane

Very strong quick drying glue in hollow of cane

Xsection

TED'S FOAM RUBBER HEAD

gather top.

Pinch nose and sew position

position for eye.

Tack at base of nose.

Tube of foam. 25 cm. circ.

Filling

gather top — gather base

flatten out pleat and sew across top

position of tack to make nose.

toymaker's eyes

white card teeth.

felt tip painted mouth.

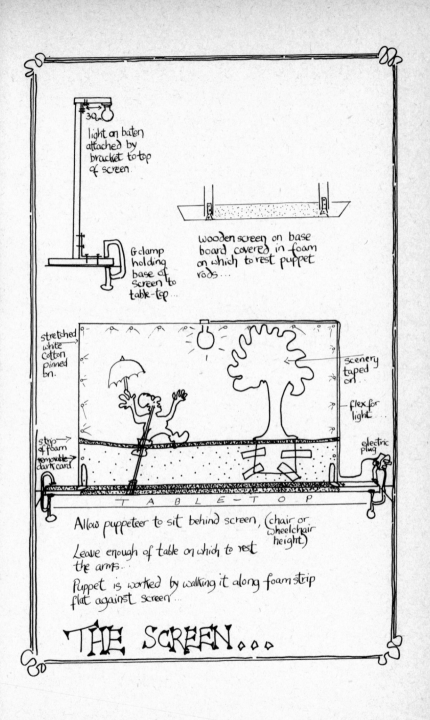

30cm

light on baten attached by bracket to top of screen.

G clamp holding base of screen to table-top...

Wooden screen on base board covered in foam on which to rest puppet rods...

stretched white cotton pinned on.

scenery taped on.

flex for light...

strip of foam
removable dark card.

electric plug

T A B L E - T O P

Allow puppeteer to sit behind screen, (chair or wheelchair height)

Leave enough of table on which to rest the arms...

Puppet is worked by walking it along foam strip flat against screen...

THE SCREEN...

The following instructions are for making puppets based on the design of historical examples.

Shadow puppetry via the overhead projector

Place a piece of clear acetate over some white paper on the projection screen. Draw a figure on the screen. Draw a figure on the acetate, remove the white paper and look at the figure as it has become visible on the viewing screen. Move the sheet around so that the figure becomes animated—add music if you like.

Next work on plain black shadow images—very figurative, simply trace them from picture books. They may need cutting and altering slightly so that the silhouettes are clean. Then put these on to the screen.

Your aim should be to encourage a handicapped person to transfer from the flat picture to the projected image and still to recognise the shapes and features of the figures. Paper drinking straw rods taped to the figures will help them to become more mobile, but initially finger contact is important.

Going on to the big shadow screen

You need a large wooden screen with plain white cotton stretched across it. The screen needs to be fixed to keep it still. A good suggestion is to put the frame on brackets which then may be G or C clamped on to a table-top (see illustration p. 63).

Now, the light source. The frame may easily be stood in front of a window in which case daylight would be the natural light source, but it is often easier to concentrate the attention of the group by working in near darkness with artificial light to illuminate the screen alone. The effect of the whole session will be much more dramatic and in essence more magical.

A light needs to be placed centrally about 300 mm (a foot) away from the screen. A bracket is used in the drawing. Some people prefer to use an angled lamp on brackets. These are good, but they swing out of positions easily and this may prove to be a disadvantage, especially when working with people who are likely to fiddle with things.

The puppets have to be worked flat against the screen. At

first, use plain black silhouette and do not joint the puppets.

The only material used in this book is black spectrum paper—it is quite thick, easily available from artist suppliers, and fine for smaller puppets. If you find the experiments successful, then move on to thicker material: card, even lino, or plywood. As you get more advanced it is important that you provide ready-made puppets yourself.

Return to the screen continually while you are making the puppets. Beware of beavering away in uncertainty: USE THE SCREEN. If you are nervous and self-conscious, work with a group of children and learn from them, steering *their* enthusiasm and helping them with the technical details.

The irresistibility of puppets will be an encouragement to you.

Making the shadow puppets (pages 66–68)
At this point we break our rule about not asking students to make their own puppets. This is an exercise you all do together. Give out black paper. Use dark crayons for drawing. Yes! Dark on dark. This will encourage your people to scrutinise the paper to find their marks. It will also discourage too much detail at this stage. It is important that you work side by side with your students, helping each other.

When you have each drawn a figure, use a punch to cut out eyes and mouths. Cut out the figure using big cuts, over-emphasising all the angles. If the legs need to move, simply cut them off and move them up on the figure to make an overlap and put a fastener through so that the limbs hang loosely. Alternatively you may stitch them on with dark thread. Keep returning to the screen, and work fast.

If any of the students are trying to make one side of the puppet the "right" side, then interrupt them. A SHADOW HAS NO BACK.

Treat moving arms the same way as the legs, but greater scope for action may be achieved by using the pattern provided.

If the pace of the session slackens, then come back to the screen for a quick "show" and encourage each other with applause. Then get back to finishing. Temporarily attach rods

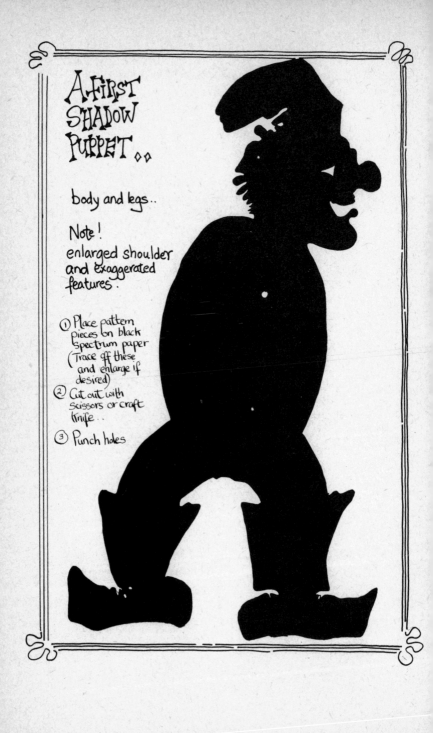

A FIRST SHADOW PUPPET ..

body and legs..

Note!
enlarged shoulder
and exaggerated
features.

① Place pattern
pieces on black
Spectrum paper
(Trace off these
and enlarge if
desired)

② Cut out with
scissors or craft
knife..

③ Punch holes

A FIRST SHADOW PUPPET

arm pattern...

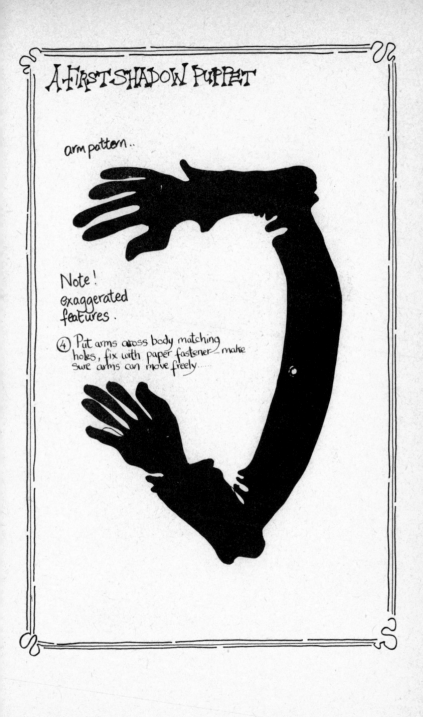

Note!
exaggerated
features.

④ Put arms across body matching
holes, fix with paper fastener. make
sure arms can move freely......

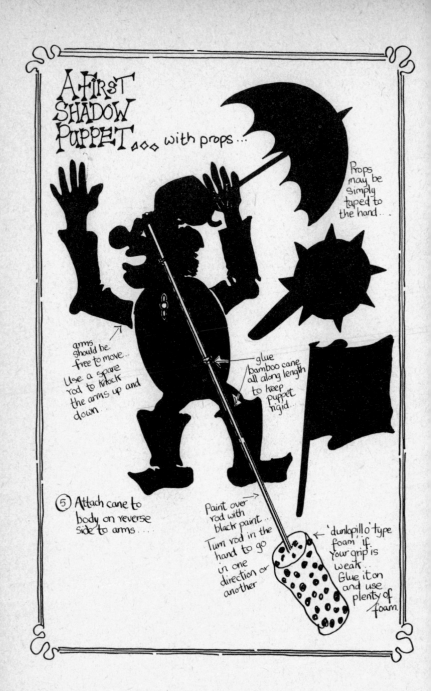

A FIRST SHADOW PUPPET... with props...

Props may be simply taped to the hand...

arms should be free to move...
Use a spare rod to knock the arms up and down.

glue bamboo cane all along length to keep puppet rigid...

⑤ Attach cane to body on reverse side to arms....

Paint over rod with black paint... Turn rod in the hand to go in one direction or another

'dunlopillo' type foam' if your grip is weak.. Glue it on and use plenty of foam.

to puppets with a plastic adhesive such as 'Blu-tak'. Whatever happens during the session END EVERY SESSION WITH A SHORT PERFORMANCE, even if it is as simple as making the puppets dance to music.

You may be wondering why it is that I recommend breaking the rule, and starting with an outline session on the making of shadow puppets. The point is that shadow puppets are made in this case of very limited materials, and you are working to a clear drawn pattern so the problem of materials "turning into other things" does not arise. These puppets will only ever be black paper on sticks. The observer as well as the puppeteer can thus be objective and detached: the puppets are telling a story and you are using them as moving pictures, to illustrate.

If you are able to work with other people around you, it is a good thing for the students to see you grow close to a three-dimensional puppet while you are creating him. Take for example the Tubby puppet. You have given him a name, so when anyone wants to know what you are doing you are making a Tubby puppet. You and your puppet are providing a focus for activity. Perhaps someone can hold something for you while you glue it. It is all staged—plan every step with certain objectives: to find out who is going to be interested, who needs more encouragement, who *can* make something and who will enjoy being part of the group as a spectator. And being a spectator is not a bad thing. Just a short time with this group, and then on another occasion you might bring out the puppet again and do a little more on him.

See how the group are affected and how much they remember of what was done last time. And also look out for the questions. Get your relationship with the puppet established: "Tubby puppet, my friend—at least he will be when he's finished."

Another puppet effectively made in public is the sock puppet. Why? Well, he takes character very quickly indeed. Follow the instructions and you will see. The first thing that happens is his mouth, which means he can say "hello", eat, have a cuddle, steal, pinch and snap—not bad for one and a

A CHARACTER : TUBBY..

(dual control puppet)

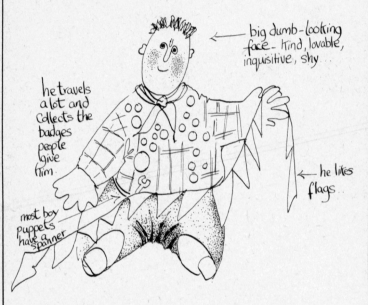

← big dumb-looking face - kind, lovable, inquisitive, shy...

he travels a lot and collects the badges people give him.

← he likes flags..

most boy puppets have a spanner

He also has in his pocket; a puppet frog, tadpole, spider, a peanut, a balloon, a clockwork gorilla and a picture of a witch painted by a boy who had been in the audience -

It is important to make every puppet special by adding special details to show his character...

Details can be added and the puppet completed as a group activity..

A SOCK PUPPET..

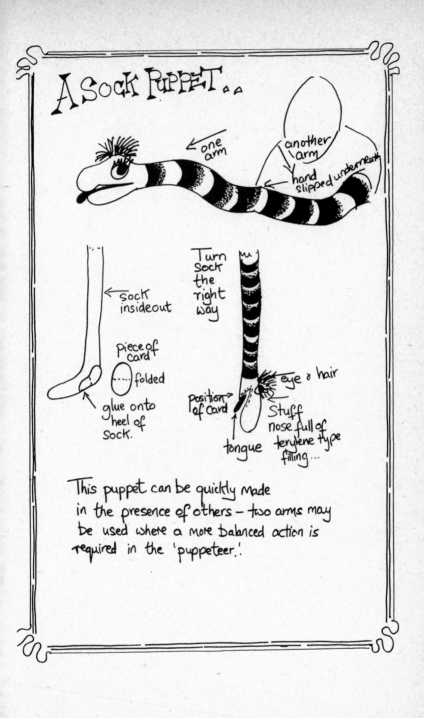

one arm

another arm

hand slipped underneath

sock insideout

Turn sock the right way

Piece of card

folded

glue onto heel of sock.

position of card

eye & hair

Stuff nose full of terylene type filling...

tongue

This puppet can be quickly made in the presence of others – two arms may be used where a more balanced action is required in the 'puppeteer.'

half minutes' work! Fill his nose with stuffing and then he can sniff; add eyes and hair and he is complete. Large and small people like these puppets, so take extra socks: you may end up making several.

When making three-dimensional puppets it is easy to over-decorate and so take away from the integrity of the puppet. Always ask the question: Why am I adding this or that? What does it tell me about the character? If sticking this bit of ribbon here or that bit of braid there in fact tells you nothing about the character but something about your tendency to meddle, leave it out. Always remember that in the end you are building a character to whom you are to relate. In making the puppet you have the chance to get inside him, and to get to know him especially well. Your knowledge will affect the way you work and handle the puppet.

We have looked at some methods of making puppets, but there are many others and I hope that anyone reading this will be encouraged to discover ways for himself. The aim in all puppet-making should be to make something which when animated will become an exciting and stimulating character. Making the puppet is just the beginning of a longer process as the personality of the puppet emerges.

A note on junk puppetry
Sometimes it is appropriate to use a variety of quickly made puppets from junk (old containers—boxes, cartons, etc). Be prepared to dispose of them. They are often unable to take the strain of involuntary or ungentle movement, and break up easily. So treat them as junk and be prepared to throw them out at the end of a session (first salvaging the re-usable parts). It is very easy to get buried under rubbish, which is what these puppets are . . . but just as the beachcomber on the beach can find *some* use for *some* of the things washed up, so there is *some* use for junk puppets. As an initial introduction to puppets or as a way of understanding animation, junk puppetry has a place in experiment. However, this kind of puppetry should not be used as an alternative to making puppets that are thought out, well made and a true expression of creativity.

PART TWO

Puppetry as a Performing Art

The audience and what takes place there
The puppet character in special therapy

Puppetry as a Performing Art

The audience and what takes place there

IF puppetry as an art had to depend on the hundreds of papier-maché heads drying on classroom windowsills, or on the procrastinating teachers whose children go through the school gates with the just-finished dolls just before term ends with never a performance behind them, then puppetry would well and truly have been rubbed out of history. But as it is, puppetry has remained elusive, and out of the hands of the educationalists, has retained its primitive magic . . . almost exclusively in the power of the performer. Although attempts have been made by bands of enthusiastic amateurs to make puppets respectable by dragging them into the camps of education or even psychology, they have resisted domestication.

Recently an ancient university hired a Punch and Judy man during the examination period to perform to the students after breakfast. Should we despise the puppeteer for providing—dare we say it—a diversion? At the other extreme an International Conference on Puppets and Therapy made a determined effort to be serious by talking its way through a weekend, struggling from one specialist jargon to the next before dwindling away into confusion as one person after another announced that she had in fact given up puppetry with people who were mentally handicapped. It was a very "sensible" business until someone had the wit actually to produce a puppet—a suitcase full of them, in fact . . . a reminder that there are some things impossible to measure—(why *do* we laugh and cry at puppets?).

But how does one define the emotional climate of art? How does one classify the emotions which give rise to the experience of beauty? If you leaf through textbooks of experimental pyschology, you won't find much of it. When Behaviourists use the word "emotion", they nearly always refer to hunger, sex, rage and fear and the related effects of the release of adrenalin. They have no explanation to offer for the curious reaction one experiences when listening to Mozart, or looking at the ocean, or reading for the first time John Donne's Holy Sonnets. Nor will you find in the textbooks a description of the physiological processes accompanying the reaction: moistening of the eyes, catching one's breath, followed by a kind of rapt tranquillity, the draining of all tensions . . .

(from *The Ghost in the Machine*, Arthur Koestler)

Dorothy, a woman of about 30, severely subnormal and totally blind, came to see a show. She depended on the reactions of all those around her, also severely or profoundly handicapped. But she sat listening intently. The first show was a shadow show. "Lovely, it were lovely," she murmured, wrapped up in the experience. Throughout the performance the whole group had watched in *silent* concentration. But obviously what was happening in the audience had been richly communicative.

What *does* happen in the audience?

The performance throws out hints of reality suggested by the performer, according to her view of it. The puppets are the medium for the message. Those in the audience use their imaginative powers to construct a full picture in relation to themselves. The activity does not stop there, however. They then communicate to others what they are experiencing so that they too share in the whole event. Perhaps they communicate by in some way *overflowing* in their own experience rather than by a conscious "I will tell the person sitting next to me." The power to transpose the symbolic into the real experience through the imagination will be stronger in some than in others; but the desire to communicate will override the handicap and that desire to share will draw a group together into a harmony out of which healing in the social sense is available.

Lisa, a girl who was severely mentally handicapped and also usually very slow to react because of the effect of heavy

drugging, became so alert during the show that she responded
to a performer by giving her name and went up close to a
screen to point at the puppet moving around—and said, quite
correctly, "Bird!" Later during another show, she recognised
the scenery and said in a loud voice "Flower!"

David came to the show with a few other children from his
school and some very protective teachers, who were unwilling
to let these children from a school for severely handicapped
children mix with "normal" children in the audience.
Gradually the longing in David to become more actively
involved overcame obedience as slowly he crept forward to get
nearer the performers. He was given a musical instrument to
play and an incredible look of delight spread across his face as
he discovered a demand that was about to be made of him and
he waited for his cue—the cue to share.

"Oh, where's my poor little Gretel?" sang out Peter in
despair.

"I don't know, dearie!" came the reply from Molly in the
audience.

"I like sausages, big fat juicy sausages!" sang Punch.

"We like sausages, big fat juicy sausages!" came the echo
from the audience led by one who held a continuous
conversation with the puppets:

"You bad, Mister Punch."

"Oh no I'm not!"

"You *bad*, Mister Punch. Look who's coming. Policeman!
There's Mister Punch, Mister Policeman! No, he's gone
now—that way! No! Behind you! Look he *there*: He had the
stick! Oh, *naughty bad* Punch. He's dead—you bad, Mister
Punch."

and so on to the end:

"If I promise to be a good boy will you let me help the
Queen?"

"No!"

"If . . ."

"No! You *bad*, Mister Punch!"

"But if I *promise*!"

"No—you *bad*, Mister Punch!"

and on that occasion Punch ignominiously retired to the nether regions collected by the Devil Puppet in response to public demand!

In a play with a baby:

"I'm going to steal the baby!"
Howls from the audience "Oh no! Get off the baby! Leave the baby! Bad man, bad man! Poor baby."

In another play, a King gives the girl away to the wicked Magician. The audience picked up on a previous idea and shouted, "Put him in the dustbin!"
To which the King replied singing,

"All I want is more gold!
  All I want is more gold!
  More and more and more and more and more gold!"

And the audience replied "All I want is more gold! All I want is more gold! Put him in the dustbin? Spank his bottom!"

The hero has lost his girl: "I've lost my poor little Gretel!"
"Oh!"
"I've lost my poor little Gretel!"
"Oh!"
"I've lost my poor little Gretel!"
"Oh!"
"I don't know where she's gone."

These are illustrations not of how an audience is *expected* to act, but of how on different occasions, different audiences, or members of audiences *have* acted wonderfully spontaneously and to such a high degree of involvement that the interjections seem scripted. Such involvement could not occur without a comparatively high level of understanding, imaginative interpretation and the ability to communicate with others in the audience. It is important to recognise that there are occasions when people, even the profoundly handicapped, can exceed the usual expectations of them.

In these examples, teachers and care staff responded to the

reactions of the audiences with surprise and pleasure. They were able to observe that:

1. The play does not have to "talk down" to the audience;
2. The audience had demonstrated comprehension of the events in the drama;
3. The audience had operated as a whole (rather than as many individuals, which is more common amongst those who are mentally handicapped);
4. That characters had been recognised and moral choices made by the audience on the basis of what they personally knew about the characters' values.

Audience reaction is often inexplicable, it is part of the whole mystery of our response to art. Although behaviourists try to pin reactions down to physiological occurrences, they cannot explain *why* we respond as we do. In the same way we must be prepared to be surprised at what might happen in an audience of people who are mentally handicapped, and to acknowledge the expression of pleasure or sadness or any other appropriate emotion as valuable. Entertainment as diversion need not be looked down upon (those university students had no trouble accepting puppetry as entertainment!). But the members of the International Conference were falling by the wayside in their attempts to introduce puppetry to the handicapped because they were looking *past* the evidence of reactions with puppets—an emotional reaction, a *human* reaction they were not equipped as specialists to handle (none of the Conference members who had this trouble were actually artists). They felt insecure about measuring the immeasurable.

Recently a teacher in a school for severely subnormal children said she wanted very much to include puppetry, but that she felt she ought to do something educational instead! Comments like that really do lead one to wonder whether artists are the only ones left to work sensitively with the feelings people express!

The audience situation is not passive but very active. The audience is also usually a very happy place to be. But this depends on various conditions which are nearly always external, analysed on page 80. You will notice from the Table

Table 1

Conditions for performance

Show	Venue	Lighting	Seating	Duration
Glove	Out of doors	Sunlight	Younger children on grass at front then a gap of fifteen feet to where adults were sitting on chairs.	20 min.
Glove	School canteen	Dull available light	Mainly on chairs, helpers sitting on tables with some children or amongst all the others.	45 min.
Glove	Large classroom	Artificial light	Everyone on chairs, crammed in. Special care children at front with anyone else with extra hearing or sight problems.	30 min.
Glove	Very large hall	Dull available light	All handicapped adults on chairs everyone else standing around on perimeter not watching.	30 min.
Glove	Playgroup in large room	Dull available light	On floor or on knees of helpers.	10 min.
Glove	Children's Home sitting room	Artificial light	Chairs, wheelchairs, floor and on knees of helpers.	25 min.
Glove, Show with more difficult plot.	All male hospital hall	Dull available light.	On floor.	30 min.
Glove	All female hospital hall	Dull available light	All on chairs crammed in, helpers mixed in.	30 min.
Glove	Both sexes hospital hall	Dull available light	All on chairs, crowded, helpers mixed in.	40 min.
Glove	Theatre mixed handicapped	Theatrical lighting	On chairs and floor, of long, narrow auditorium.	40 min.
Shadow	Theatre mixed handicapped	As shadow, black out.	On knees, in chairs, crowded	10 min.
Shadow	Hospital school hall	Dull light not blackout	On chairs, on knees, teachers mixed in.	10 min.

Helpers	Reaction
Few in number and uninvolved	Poor concentration, too hot and too many distractions outside. Adults too far away to focus attention, also too hot. One child very disruptive and helpers unwilling to control him—show had to stop.
Giving encouragement continuously, enjoyed reactions of children	Excellent show—good balance and play between performer and audience. Show was almost double the usual length as a result, with good concentration.
Staff tried to encourage but were not mingled	Good response but the less able needed more individual encouragement.
Were not part of the audience at all, talked throughout and hearing made difficult for handicapped.	Show curtailed and not restarted.
Very involved and trying to encourage children	Very short show as the children were too young—some cried—others unable to follow at all.
Friendly and affectionate with audience—babies to aged 16	Very good response, some children unusually responsive.
Not very involved and none in audience.	Good response but they could have gained more with help over story.
Very encouraging particularly the most popular male staff.	Very good, with good grasp of story, very excitable audience.
Very encouraging they enjoyed seeing the residents' enjoyment.	Excellent response, new bits of business added as a result of creativity of audience.
All young teenagers, unable to give very much support, but did their best.	Mixed up response—broken up through the audience. Shape of auditorium made it very hard to get a good general unified response.
Very supportive, determined that even the most profoundly handicapped should gain from the experience.	All children absolutely silent in concentration—whispers from staff only.
Teachers noisy— encouraging children	Lack of blackout meant the audience was less concentrated in their attention—but very involved.

that these differing conditions are related to the kind of space, the seating arrangements and the people who are helping. Where the helpers have not been supportive, where they have not been prepared to share the show, there has sometimes been a complete breakdown in the circle of communication: performer-individual in the audience—whole audience-performer. Sometimes people in the audience have become disruptive as a result of bad helping, and then it has been necessary actually to stop the show.

The Setting

These shows are all professional shows. The improvised glove puppet show is usually quick, fast flowing, with the maximum opportunity for audience involvement of a very basic kind; although it can become quite complex, as we have seen in the examples of performer-audience dialogue above.

The response of the audience gives an excellent opportunity for a person who is usually quiet or withdrawn to express himself under the cover of the more extrovert. The length of the improvised show depends very much upon the interaction between the performer and the audience. If the response is good, it usually means that the concentration is good as well, so extra characters can be brought on and extra business take place.

Although special lighting can enhance the action and add atmosphere, it is not entirely necessary. If the show is out of doors or there is only one light source in a room, the puppeteer usually faces the light to ensure that the audience itself is not looking into the light. If the shows can be performed in darkness except for the use of a single spotlight for a booth show, or the lit-up screen for the shadow show, this actually helps some people to concentrate their attention on the action. This is partly a response to the atmosphere but also to the fact that other potentially distracting visual stimuli have been cut out. Often the audience is better behaved in darkness too!

The seating arrangements are very important. There should be enough chairs or space for everyone to be in front of the booth. It is no good having half the people slouched around lying on the floor behind the main audience area and of course

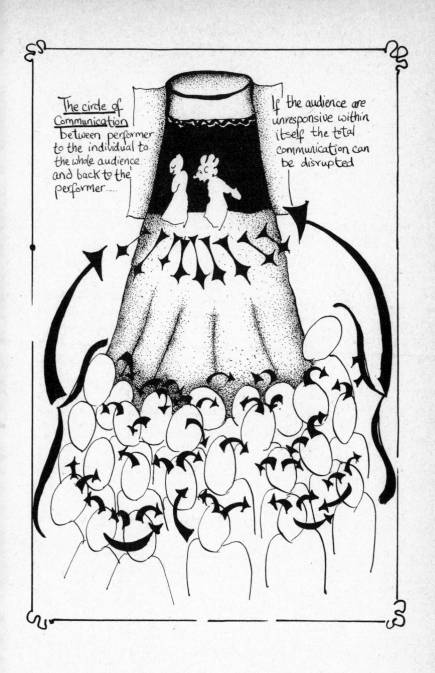

The circle of
Communication
between performer
to the individual to
the whole audience
and back to the
performer......

If the audience are
unresponsive within
itself the total
communication can
be disrupted

it is vital that helpers stay to watch the show with the rest of the audience.

I remember one performance on a very hot day in a hospital. The residents were simply parked in front of the booth by the attendants, who then deserted them. Most of the audience were in wheelchairs, and many elderly. They had all been left with ice-cream cornets in their hands, even though many could not eat without help. They watched the show alone in the sun, with melting ice-cream dribbling into their laps. In addition, there was a fairground next door, with a discotheque and loudspeakers. That afternoon was an object lesson in how to guarantee failure.

Everyone in the audience should be as close together as possible, with no unfriendly spaces! Helpers should be inter-mingled with those who need help. The responses of the helpers make a difference both to the comfort and the progress of the entire audience. Helpers should be able to give verbal support to those less able, encouraging them in any response. Some people actually need physical support: their hand held, someone to point their fingers when they want to tell the puppets something, or even someone to clap their hands for them at the end. Even those who are physically able might need the reassurance of another's presence to help them understand, or just to feel comfortable.

Helpers, in short, have to be sharing their lives and their more integrated personalities with the people with handicaps. The sharing experience of the audience in turn can be much enriched by the right supportive attitudes. And helpers who simply dismiss puppets as "childish" cannot provide such support. Recently a young musician wrote that he preferred to be with children, rather than adults, and he wished people would "grow down instead of up". What a lot a person has missed when he has "grown out" of puppets! And how hard it is to perform to an audience which thinks it is far too sophisticated to enjoy the show.

The profoundly handicapped audience
We have been describing conditions of shows for people who can be taken to see them. But there are other people who are

SEATING..

Long narrow hall
Helpers at rear –

(Difficult shape to play in : ① Poor audibility,
② Poor visibility ③ Helpers react to the
reactions of the front of the house.

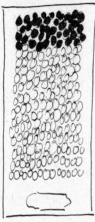

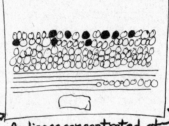

**Audience concentrated at
rear of hall.**
Reactions often slow to come.
It would be better to move
everyone forward.

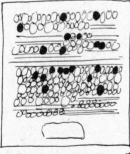

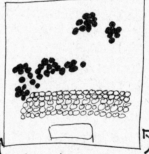

Audience scattered
with too many spaces...
is a slower audience.
Everyone moved forward,
with helpers intermingled,
would be better.

Helpers standing around
at back separate
from the main audience
have a disruptive effect.
Everyone should be sitting
down with helpers scattered
throughout.

confined to the ward of a hospital, and never come out to see a performance because they are too handicapped. In this case, we have to take our show to them. A performance in a ward for the very profoundly handicapped underlines the loving care the patients are receiving and emphasises that even for people so disabled, there is something called a life worth living.

It is interesting first to observe how such wards are run. Are there flowers around? Pictures on the walls? Is it a ward with only beds in it or are there spaces for the carriages? These wards are often cut off from outside visitors or even from other people in the hospital. The patients too are very isolated, often unable to communicate in a recognisable manner (except perhaps to those working closest to them), and heavily drugged. There seems to be little hope for any response to puppets. Where can any hope lie for the visiting performer? We may not be able to measure understanding, so we have to accept the idea of some invisible potential.

How does one perform in such unlikely circumstances? It is important first to get to know the staff, and to be prepared for them to remove patients who may become distressed. (I remember being most insulted when one by one virtually my whole audience was removed.) Always check to find out which patients you can touch with the puppets and which react badly to sudden sounds or disturbing movements. Keep to your story line and move around from one patient to the other. Perform to the most able, including the staff, whose enjoyment will infect the rest of the audience. Even the most severely handicapped will often respond to atmosphere. Include music in the performance to enrich the experience.

As an alternative to the floor show, for the most severely handicapped a shadow show to music is often appropriate. The big clear images on the screen are easy to follow and enjoyable to watch even if the storyline is lost. A shadow show using a tungsten bulb (the ordinary household kind) is easier to watch than a television screen. The way light is emitted from the television screen at a rate of fifty flickers a second can cause discomfort.

I remember one particular hospital visit with special pleasure. We went into the ward where some of the most

severely handicapped women were housed. The first
impression was very encouraging. The staff had taken great
pride in the look of the place. There were flowers and plants
everywhere—often out of reach and most of them plastic, but
they added colour. There were pictures on the walls too. As we
prepared and took out the puppets and the musical instruments
I kept looking around. It was good to see the kitchen staff and
cleaning ladies coming out as well. In the theatre, if the stage
staff stop what they are doing to listen to a performer it is a sign
that *you* are good; but from my experience of visiting hospitals
and schools, if the ancillary staff are interested in what is going
on then it is a sign that the *place* is good.

I heard a repeated scratching noise. There was a grown
woman lying under a table scraping her nails along the ridged
surface of a radiator. Another woman stood facing into a
corner moaning to herself.

Soon everyone was ready. Some of the more able "helpers"
had stayed behind after helping us to carry our equipment in.

It was very difficult for us to understand the reactions of the
residents to the puppets. They just didn't react in the same way
as we might—for example, nodding the head did not
necessarily mean "yes" and some of the patients rocked
constantly backwards and forwards, or made noises. In order
to try to get some common contact I took out a little bird
puppet which was fixed to the end of a sprung rod. I made the
girl puppet catch the bird in one hand and stroke it gently. I
asked who else would like to do the same. A positive response
would of course mean that the person must have observed and
understood what was happening between the two puppets, so I
expected only the "helpers" to respond to my invitation. But I
was amazed to see the reaction. Out of these half-aware bodies
which had been looking vaguely in my direction, rocking back
and forth, noisy in a way unrelated to anything I was doing,
unravelled hands from all over the place to appeal for the bird.
I made the bird flutter around and land on each hand to be
caressed and even kissed before fluttering on. This was a totally
unexpected demonstration of a degree of understanding among
the audience far beyond my expectations, and a lesson to me.

It is sometimes a good idea to prepare groups of people for the "big" show. This will give you an opportunity to see how much understanding of the plot and the characters to expect. When a character is known in advance the interaction between the personalities follows on naturally.

Meeting the puppets in anticipation of the main show

We were meeting several groups throughout the morning. They were brought to us in groups of six to eight. Attached to the group, but not part of it, was Penelope. She had adopted the room, but nothing would ever induce her to take part in any activity in the occupational therapy department. For months at a time she would simply occupy the corner of her favourite room. She sat there an indomitable presence. She wore an overcoat over her clothes and carried a shopping bag in which she kept various treasures which no doubt I would be seeing during the morning. I wondered if it was coincidence that brought her to the room I was in, the second year running? If I looked at her directly she became coy and thrust her hand right into her mouth. I don't recall her having teeth but I'm certain she had a jawbone—and yet her hand would go in like a rat being swallowed by a snake.

We repeated roughly the same programme for each group. I acted out the story using the puppets and as I changed puppets I handed them on to one of the group to hold. When the puppet was due to reappear then the person holding the puppet at that moment would use it—in character. The aim was that they would know what character they were holding and what part he played in the drama. We also used song and sound effects to introduce each character. There were a few deaf mutes and we encouraged them to play the drums which they did effectively enough, enjoying the rhythm, and, without realising it of course, deafening the rest of us.

After the second group had come and gone, I noticed that Penelope had moved slightly closer to the circle of chairs. She had done this inconspicuously while we were replacing the puppets. She fixed her eyes on each newcomer, daring him to come closer and then if he responded she buried herself back behind a huge well-chewed, mail-order catalogue. When I looked at her she produced a woolly hat which she pulled well

down on her head as if threatening to leave! The moment came
when I offered the little bird to the group and they put up
their hands to stroke the puppet. But Penelope—now no
novice—pursed her rubbery lips and KISSED the bird before
allowing it to be passed on. She had been watching all the time!
She retired back into her corner in triumph—she had showed
'em all.

Later on in the afternoon, I performed the show for the
whole occupational therapy department, in the traditional
manner from the booth. At the end of the show I was inside the
booth still clearing up after a very good performance. I jumped
suddenly as someone pinched my bottom. I tore back the
curtain, expecting to see one of the men there, only to find
Penelope, who gave me a thumbs-up sign and a big grin before
shuffling away with her woolly hat down low over her eyes and
her shopping bag bulging at her side. I think she had had a
good day!

Referring back to the check list for assessment
The assessment points should be used from both the audience's
point of view and the performer's.

The group work already described had been structured to
make these points objectives:

1. *That a person should be able to relate to the puppet.*
2. That he should be able to fulfil his obligations to show the
puppet to others.
3. That he should be able to rise to the expectations of others
as they show the desire to see him perform.
4. That he should be able to *extend his social repertoire:
communication, intellectual content, expressions of feelings, the ability
to make moral choices.*
5. That he should be able to make the appropriate actions
with the puppet.
6. That he should be able to *develop sensitivity to the performance
situation.*

The italicised points are those where the audience is as active
as the performer, and where the audience has objectives to
achieve.

All these criteria are based on the person's ability to understand what is happening, not solely on an emotional response.
As you have seen from the illustrations there can in the most
unpromising situations be a surprising degree of comprehension of the characters and the way they interact to make up
the drama. Human dignity depends to an extent on the way we
are able to allow for the possibility of being surprised in this
way, and to ascribe understanding to each person.

Exercises for the audience.
1. Place puppets on chairs and play recognition games.
"Run to Tubby", "Run to Ted!"
Invent very simple songs and catch-phrases for each
character and teach the audience to sing the correct one or
say the correct one on sight.
Teach the audience to recognise the moral character of each
puppet and to make some sign of recognition—booing,
hissing, clapping etc.
2. Call out for a person to perform with the puppets and
show your own anticipation—teach them to show their
anticipation and excitement too about seeing a puppeteer
work.
3. Teach the audience to shout out to the puppets to "help"
them make decisions. Teach clapping, "look behind you",
"look up" and so on.
4. Teach the audience ways of matching up to the mood of
the drama at any time.

The puppet character in special therapy
We have been looking at the way a visiting puppeteer might
best put on a performance before a group. However, if
puppetry is to be a valuable part of the occupational resources
for a mentally handicapped person, there should be day to day
back-up sessions in the usual manner of therapy. Many
therapists are already using puppets in one-to-one situations or
in small group work.
When watching an audience, it is sometimes quite
disturbing to see people usually quiet or withdrawn come to life
in a very open and often emotional way. I have heard people

declare that they had stopped using puppets because they could not control the very positive reactions they were getting from some patients: seeing such audience reaction can frighten therapists off from using puppets at all. Yet it is in this very reaction that the great therapeutic power of puppetry lies.

The important things to remember are to have very definite treatment aims, and to recognise puppetry as art. The latter is helped first of all by making sure you have a beautiful selection of puppets, full of character and stimulating to watch and work.

A letter from a speech therapist

May I just say again how much I enjoyed your day's demonstration and lecture at our college. I felt very encouraged and some of your enthusiasm has rubbed off on me. I was particularly interested by the way you used a puppet to be alongside a child doing a difficult or potentially boring bit of work, to gain a better response. I tried this when I got back here with a sleeve puppet which I'd already used in some sessions, a caterpillar called Henry. I've started using him regularly with certain children, watching what they're doing, inspecting their work and copying from them in his own book—à la Hilary Witch. I've also tried to develop his personality and looks—he wears glasses for reading—and I found that children respond with more interest and spontaneous back-chat. A little boy this morning asked Henry if he'd noticed anything different about him! He'd had a haircut.

The whole thing is great fun—but I take your point about "making a child excited does not necessarily mean that he is learning" so am bearing this in mind and trying not to lose sight of my treatment aims. It can sometimes be a failing, I think, in a therapist if you like a piece of equipment so much you can begin to use it less discriminately, fitting the activity to the equipment rather than the other way around . . .

Thank you again for passing on your enthusiasm and giving me fresh ideas . . .

This letter serves as an introduction to our starting point: the character of the puppet. Our objective is to enable a person to relate to the puppet . . . MAKE FRIENDS.

These are recorded conversations using puppets. They involve one or more persons (clients) and the puppeteer (therapist).

Tubby

This is my friend Tubby. Say "hello", Tubby. Yes *more* people. Whenever he comes out of his case there's a new person here! Shall we look at him? Yes, he's fat, isn't he? Can you guess what he collects? Yes, badges—he collects badges. He's got them all over his shirt, hasn't he? What does this one say? "The Great Milk Rush" . . . that's to remind him to drink milk. Oh, and this one says—"My name is Tubby" that's his name—Tubby. What's your name? John? Well, John, we're very pleased to meet you, aren't we Tubby? Tubby—I'll shake you! We're very pleased to meet John, AREN'T WE? Look, John, he's nodding his head. Now what other badges are there? Can you see any others that you like? That one? "Strike Gold at Eldorado". That's a bright one there—"Dales Bible Week" . . . Tubby goes all over the place with me. We've been to Switzerland, France, Canada. When we went to Canada we got off the plane and found that the captain had lost our luggage . . . all I had was Tubby and my toothbrush! Here's Tubby's toothbrush in his pocket. But we had a great time over there after we got our luggage back—and some children gave us a whole lot of badges—and . . . THIS is a balloon full of Canadian air . . . there's still a bit left in there—most of it has leaked out . . . Here's another balloon—it was a Christmas present to Tubby from Auntie Joan. Do you want me to help you blow it up, Tubby?

There . . . blow . . . blllooww and there it is . . . Oh WHOOSH! It's gone . . . the balloon has whooshed. Can you find it, John? Oh, there it is! Shall we try again? Come on, Tubby—I'm supposed to be helping you not doing all the work. You always leave me to do all the work. Let's try it again! Blllloooow. What's that, John? You *want* us to let it

go? Do you like that? All right then . . . and off it
goes—WHOOSH! Go and fetch it.

I wonder what else there is in Tubby's pocket?

Do you collect things in your pocket too John? You do? And
are they all precious things? Treasures? Oh Tubby—you are
bad. I've told you to get rid of this. Do you know what this is,
John? It's a horrible old sticky sweet. A little girl in Canada
gave it to him and he won't get rid of it. And what's this?
Listen, can you hear anything if I shake it? It's a peanut and
you can hear the peanut rattling inside the shell. Tubby likes
peanuts. One day I expect he will eat it for his dinner. What do
you like to eat for dinner?

What's this thing here? It's a picture. Can you see what it is?
A witch? Hmm that's what it looks like. A little boy painted
that and then sent it to Tubby. Tubby keeps it in his pocket.
Here's a spanner in case our car breaks down. And here are
Tubby's pets. Here's a spider. And here's a frog . . . What
does a frog do? It j . . . jumps that's right. It's going to jump
right over to you—catch . . . What do frogs have? What do
they lay? . . . They lay eggs . . . and then what do the eggs
turn into? Hang on a minute . . . He's got one just
here—that's right, a tadpole! And what's this big thing—?
Ah . . . people are always trying to persuade Tubby and me
that we came from one of these . . . a monkey—well a gorilla
then? . . . That's right let's wind it up. His name is Dar-
win—sparks spit out of his mouth as he walks along. What's
that sticking out of the top of Tubby's trouser leg? Give it a
pull—a FLAG . . . Oh lots and lots of flags!

Look at all this untidy mess! Help us to put everything
back and then it's time to go.

Are you wondering what on earth was happening? Well, first of
all, the puppet is being seen in relation to the puppeteer. This
is how we learn about other people—from the way they behave
with others. What does the above piece of acting tell us about
the puppeteer? The relationship is a play relationship, of
course. The puppeteer has a puppet who has a name and does
naughty things like hiding old sweets in his pocket. The puppet

was being very good, doing as he was told and he seemed to enjoy being with the puppeteer. He was sharing what was in his pocket—*correction*, *they* were sharing with the person in the room with them, John. Gradually even the most reticent person is drawn into this kind of scene. There is no pressure, you see, one cannot help thinking that the conversation with the puppet would have been going on anyway. There is something *"real"* about the relationship. In this little scene the "friendship" between the puppeteer and his puppet hints at reality. The other person, the "audience", uses his imaginative powers to construct a full picture in relation to himself. Thus the lines of communication spring up naturally between all three. Of course it is really between the puppeteer and the other person, the puppet is a catalyst. You have come to an unspoken agreement that you will both communicate through the puppet. For this to work the puppet has to be attractive—to both people—before we can start to treat him as if he were *real*.

Ted
(Using him with children or adults as with Tubby)

Hello, this is Ted. Ted doesn't speak. I've brought him along because he says he's worried. Do you know what he's worried about? He's worried about what goes on behind all these closed doors . . . inside these little rooms. I said one day I'd show him. And since then he's worried and worried and wanted to come in and see for himself . . .

What does happen when you come into these rooms . . . what secrets do you have? What secret things do you get up to? So here he is. And now he's here, he's NERVOUS. He doesn't have anything to be nervous about, does he? Oh look he's hiding his face—he doesn't have to do that, does he? You all like him, don't you? There's nothing for him to worry about, is there? Tell him you are all friends and then he'll be all right. There's nothing for you to worry about, you see, Ted, don't cry, here's your hanky, wipe your face . . . there, all better now.

Oh he's standing up: Isn't he tall . . .? He's so tall some people are afraid of him. But he's so quiet really and so nervous that we have to speak very very quietly when he's around or else he'll jump. Let's be very very quiet, shall we? Can you whisper, "hello" to him?

What's that? Oh, he wants to see what you have there . . . Can you put it into his hand? . . . Look he's holding out his hand. Can you bring him something else to look at? That's lovely—what is it? A little fire-engine. Whoops, you've pushed over those pegs. Give them one by one to Ted and he can help you clear up—it was partly his fault . . . Give him all the red ones first . . . that's right . . . and where are the yellow ones? That's it . . . all tidy now? Can we come back another day?

Notice some important things in this scene. The puppet needs sympathy, he is the weakest member of the group. Like Tubby he can't speak. If there is no response from the group, he can go on with the scene—it does not depend on the reaction of the audience, there is no pressure. There are however very positive invitations to become involved with the puppet.

"What do you all do in the little rooms?"

"You all like him, don't you?"

"We have to speak very quietly when he's around or else he'll jump." (This could be taken by some people as an invitation actually to make the puppet jump!)

The request to make the smallest possible noise is often a way of encouraging a first response—the smallest possible demand is often returned tenfold.

I wonder how many people are also worried about going for special therapy? This Ted has a personality that most people will recognise. He is a compulsive worrier. He needs people in the room to calm him down. If there is to be a response to this puppet it must be to satisfy the need of the character in character. Usually children and adults become engrossed with him and his problems. The key once again is to have a puppet who has a life history. And then from that point the agreement is made between the people present that they will treat the puppet as if he were real.

The puppet in a classroom

Claire, who is the puppeteer in this case, is diplegic, her legs being more affected than her arms. She is in a wheelchair but she can drag herself along the floor. Her hands are weak and shaky, especially when she makes the effort to do anything requiring precision. In addition to motor handicap there is some intellectual impairment and there are perceptual disorders.

Claire at the age of twelve can manage simple tasks such as washing up, and drying dishes, roughly laying the table. Claire finds difficulty in relating to other children—she gets over-excited and hysterical. Usually she spends time alone rocking backwards and forwards in her cold bedroom listening to her radio. Claire likes puppets.

Claire was asked if she would mind helping a puppet who was having trouble with her lessons. This advance preparation was important, it gave Claire a tremendous feeling of self-esteem because she was sharing a secret. She knew that Hilary the Green Witch was coming to share her special lesson. (The reassurance she did require was that Hilary was a *puppet* and not a real witch!) From the moment Claire possessed this basic information she happily and excitedly entered into the role of collaborator. If this child never played, rarely enjoyed the company of the other children and could seldom be persuaded to share anything, would she be able to use the puppet?

The puppet is just a puppet

The class was at work when I arrived. There was not a great deal of response from the children as a group, but Claire looked sideways at Hilary nervously.

Hilary was introduced to each child and then in return for their attention they were shown how she worked as a puppet. The children were curious about her lack of voice. It was explained to them that puppets only have the voices that real people lend them. One or two of them made "creaky" noises and I told them that was the way it was done. No attempt was made to make Hilary into a mystery—the children had to have control of the situation. It would be their imaginations doing the work, their willingness to speak through the puppet and hear through the puppet which would take them into the world of magic.

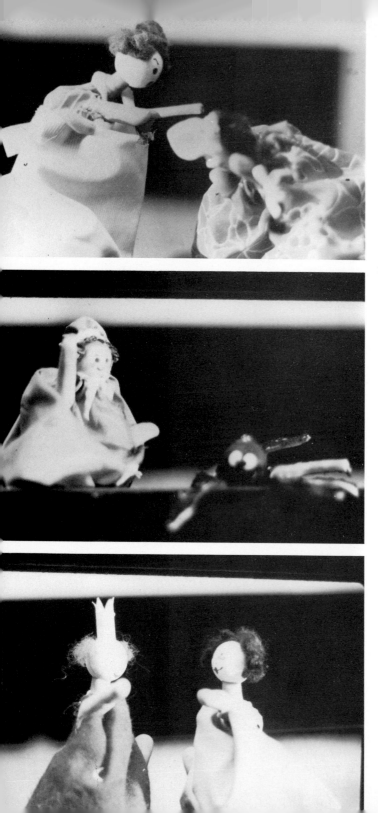

Finger puppets
are most
interesting when
filmed—either as
stills or video or
ciné.
The recorded
puppets may
then be produced
to stimulate
more work or as
a reward for past
work.
These puppets
are only finger
puppets but they
do utilize the
whole hand and
so can handle
simple props.

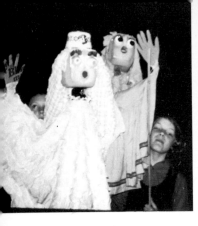

Large rod puppets – note plastic
container heads.

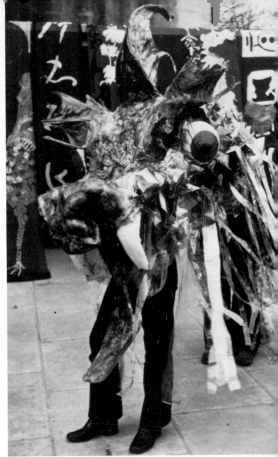

Huge dragon puppets to be worked
by two or more people in or out of
wheel chairs.

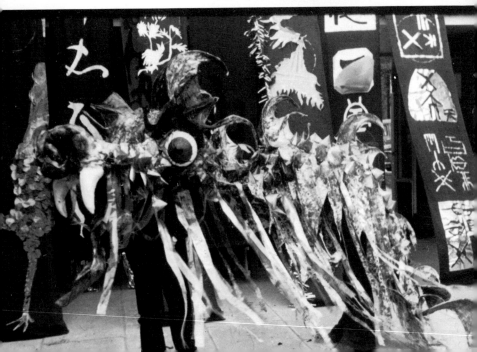

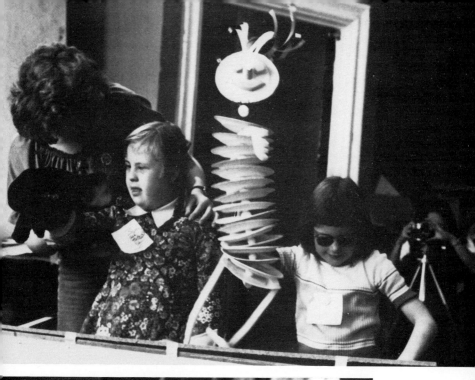

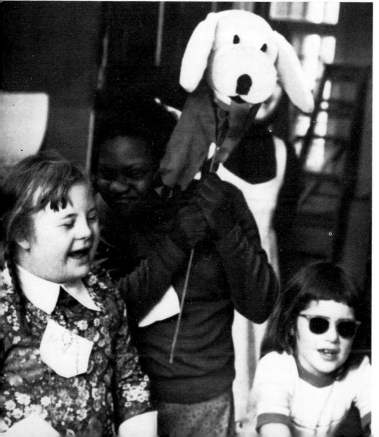

Puppetry
provides a
means for
working
and
sharing
together

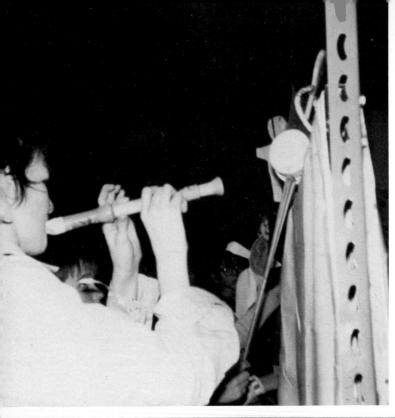

. . . and pooling all gifts

. . . and really letting go! Bringing the puppet to life is to animate it.

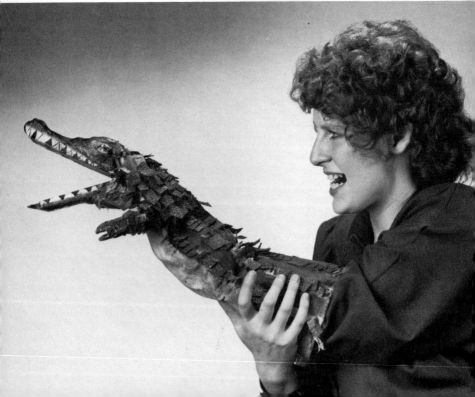

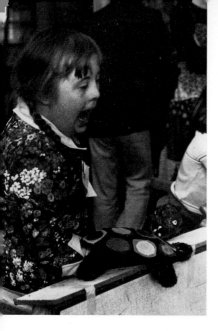

Puppetry is not only moving the puppet about but is acting with the imagination too.

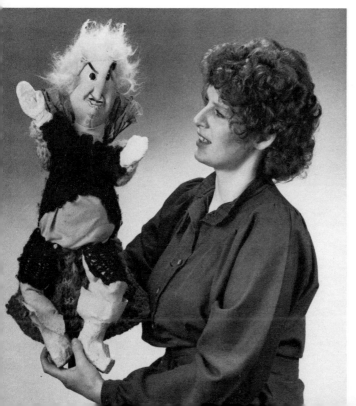

Character develops primarily from how the puppet looks – what does the appearance tell you about him?

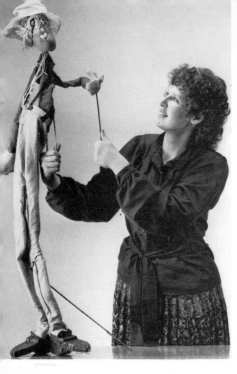

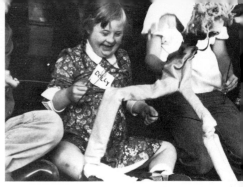

Above: Dolly, a Downes child, working the puppet with her therapists.

Left: Some people are afraid of putting their hand inside a puppet, so a rod puppet where the hand is visibly controlling the action would be more appropriate.

Below left: The puppet and puppeteer must appear to have a relationship.

Below: The relationship between the puppet and puppeteer attracts others to become involved as audience or to actually try to work the puppet themselves.

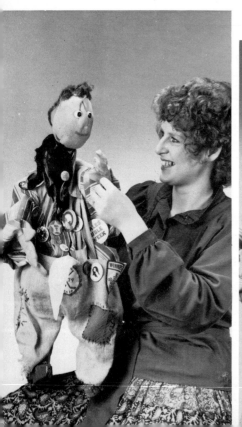

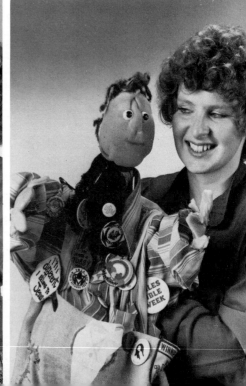

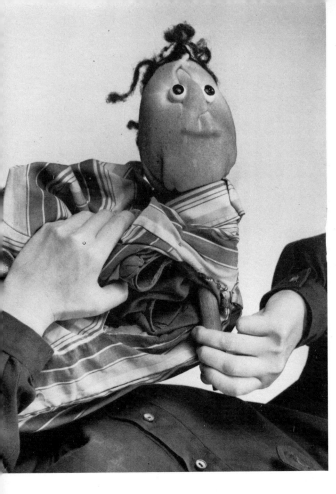

This Tubby puppet is designed for one person to hold the head-rod and another to work the hands – working together could give a more nervous person confidence.

Below left: But these puppets made by a boy severely sub-normal and with muscular dystrophy are attached to springs so the maximum movement ensues from the minimum physical effort.

Below: Plenty of action here . . .

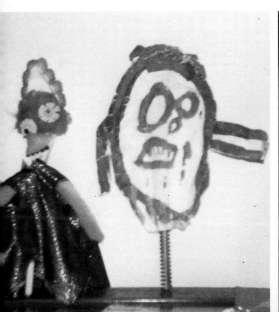

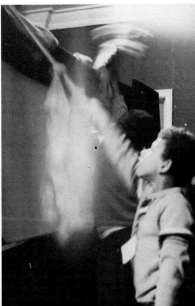

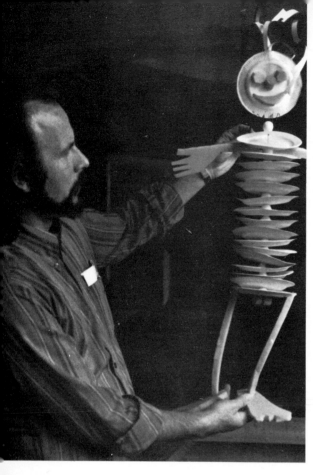

The student has designed a puppet to be used where someone has little controlled movement. The action of the puppet comes from the strong thread passing right through the paper plate/polystyrene ball body. Added pleasure comes from the head made from two plates stuck together filled with dried peas so that it rattles.

This puppet has a different expression on each side of its head. Designed for someone in a wheel chair, the centre rod simply wedges between the knees and is spun around.

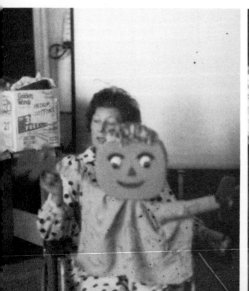

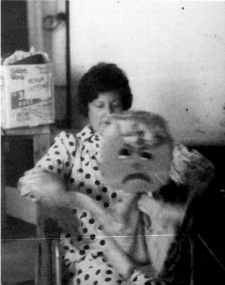

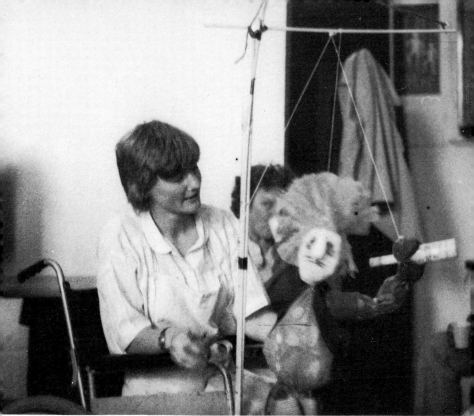

Above: Punk with bottle – the student works the puppet from a wheelchair. The control is a rubber ball threaded on to wire.

Right: Loosely jointed marionette on string attached to a cane which is springy. This was a student's solution to the problem of how to achieve the most movement in the puppet with the minimum of manipulation for someone with a physical handicap.

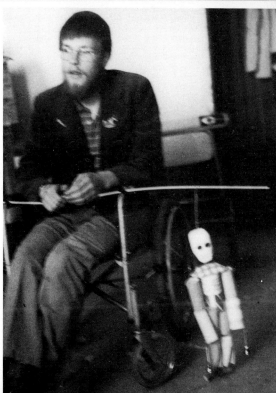

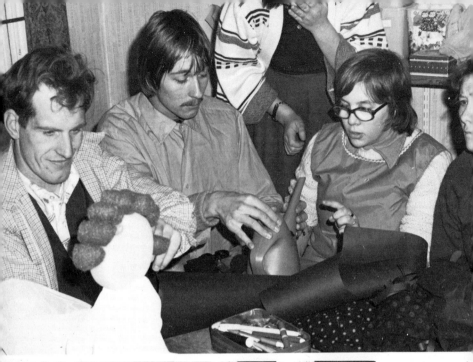

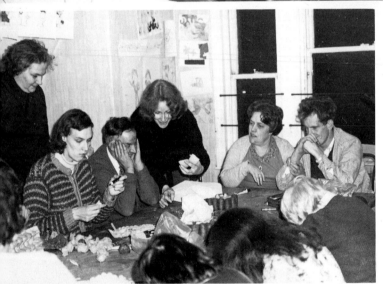

A group of mentally handicapped adults working together to make some puppets for a performance the same evening.

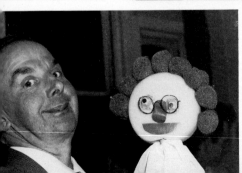

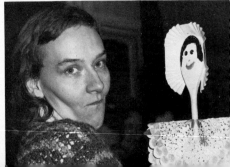

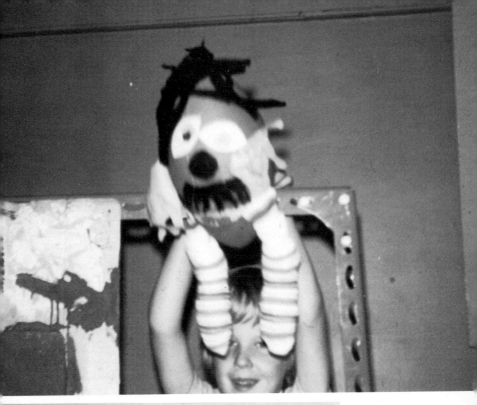

Above:
Mr Humpty:
we chose a
rugby ball for
surprise value
as it hit the
ground!

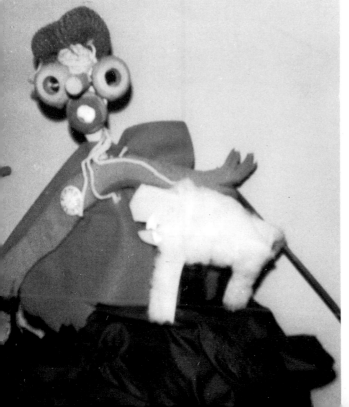

Puppets made
by an autistic
child. Mr
Nosey and
Snowy the dog.

Body image: SIMON copyright design Charig Puppets, Harrogate.

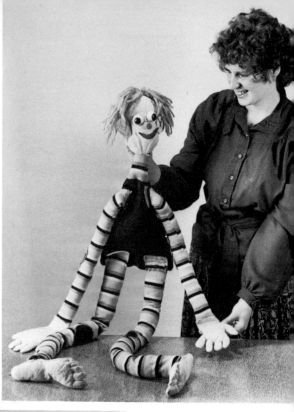

Note size of the puppet.

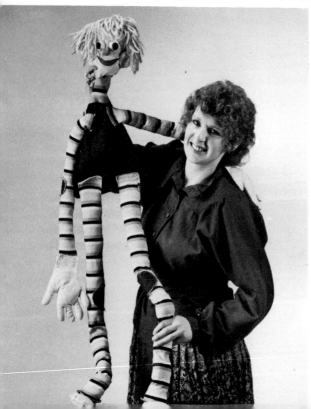

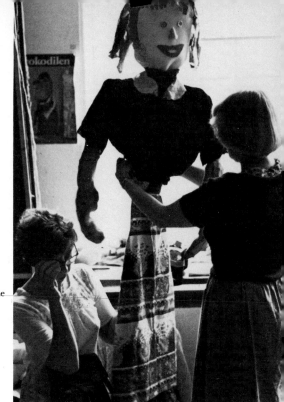

t puppets made by students to examine the image problem for adults.

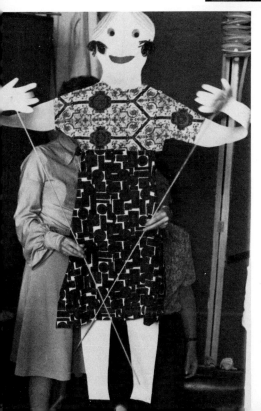

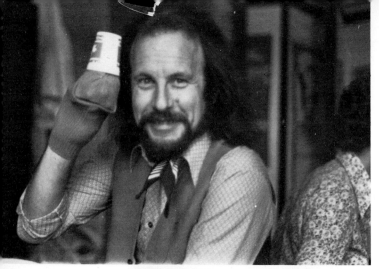

A mouth puppet – the students were asked to design puppets to draw the attention to the mouth for speaking and eating.

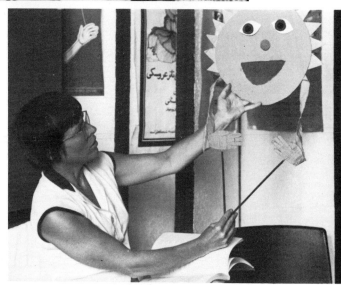

Another mouth puppet made by a student.

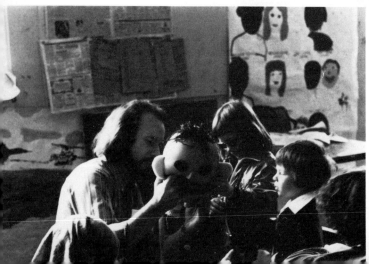

Showing the children how the puppet works.

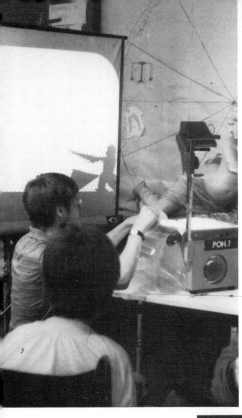

The overhead projector is useful for animating 'Bliss symbols'.

. . . or for shadow puppets.

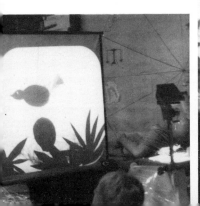

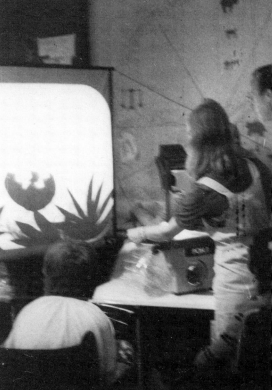

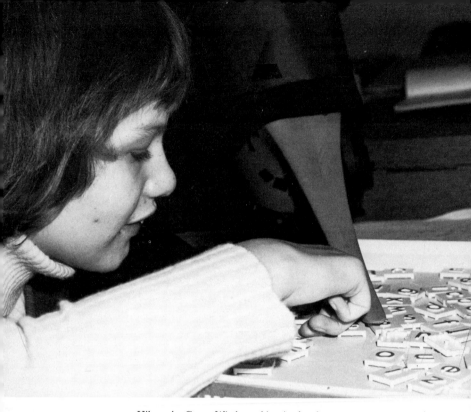

Hilary the Green Witch working in the classroom.

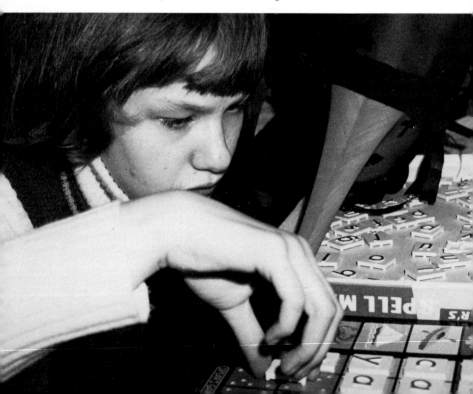

In the meantime Claire was swelling visibly with pride because Hilary was coming to work with *her*! Hilary looked over Claire's shoulder as the child carried out her work. It was a literacy exercise in which she had to read a word and then, out of a mass of letters, sort the ones she needed to make up the word and fix the letters in the right order into a peg board. The task was taxing her hand-eye co-ordination, her figure-ground perception as well as her ability to recognise words and individual letters.

It was time for Hilary to take her share of the work. Claire took Hilary on to her left hand and used the long nose of the puppet to point out the letters she needed. Claire was forced to use both hands (usually she used only her left hand, and then the whole of her body on the right side would just slump). Although large, the puppet was very light; but it needed proper handling. Claire's posture improved as she used her right hand for all the precise work, while Hilary had to "read" out each word and look at each letter as Claire held it up for her.

In this example we are moving away from the art of the puppet as we have so far envisaged it. The audience hardly mattered. But Claire actually *played* the part of teacher to Hilary, even though play was not usually part of her everyday life. Without the obligation placed on her to rise to our expectations of seeing the puppet, would she in fact have played in this way—concentrating for such a length of time? (Second point on our checklist.) Dramatically not much was going on, but certainly there was genuine identification with the puppet, in the imaginary teacher-pupil relationship.

Although no attempt was made at theatricality (so often people mean by this a superficial whipping up of the emotions), the children were still prepared by an act of the will to suspend their disbelief and thus, in the spirit of true creativity, Hilary became a stimulus for work rather than a distraction. One other boy remarked a few days later that he liked the Witch and wanted her to work with him the following day.

The ability to fantasise is a vital part of our creativity. Claire would usually have found it impossible. Using the puppet, her achievements in the classroom were increased and her behaviour much improved. It was interesting to see her moving from fantasy back to reality and back again to fantasy—in the way that children do in imaginative play in order to readjust their point of view and ensure the basic truth of their explorations. The puppet is seen here to take the pressure out of the learning situation, just as Tubby and Ted did out of the therapy one.

Although work has been done in child psychiatry, using anonymous heads and bodies as puppets, with people who are mentally handicapped, especially if they lack much imagination it is better to use puppets that are highly figurative and full of character: caricature figures in fact.

Here is an example of such puppets in action.

Sally is a large child, physically mature and ungainly, aged eleven. She was refusing to walk. Some of the teachers in the special unit thought she might be regressing to attract attention, as her mother had just had another child (the only one apart from Sally). She was severely subnormal with very little speech, no one knowing exactly how much.

The child was asked if she would like a story. She nodded excitedly as she had seen me using the puppets with other children. We went into a tiny box-like mini-classroom on wheels, and in the quiet I started to use the puppets. As it had been suggested that Sally's problems might be due to resentment towards the new baby in the family, I devised a scene which included a new baby to see how Sally would react.

Mister Punch is asleep. He wakes up and calls for Judy as he is hungry. She has no time for him as she is busy with her new baby. Punch sulks and then in a fit of rage collapses on the ground and refuses to get up again. He wants to crawl like a baby too. Judy tells him not to be so silly and then goes off to the shops leaving the baby in Punch's care. Punch hits the baby and then throws him away. A policeman comes along carrying the baby. He is cross with Punch and threatens to put Mister Punch into prison unless he gets up and promises not to hurt the baby again. Punch promises. Judy returns and kisses Punch and they dance together.

The little performance at the table lasted only ten minutes at the most, in which time Sally's attention was completely held. She became so involved that at the end of the story, she interrupted by standing up, pushing the table away and then dancing on the spot with me (and the puppets). (Usually she could be forced to her feet only by two helpers dragging her upright; on this occasion the initiative came from Sally herself.)

Her reactions to the characters on the table in front of her demonstrated complete comprehension of the story. She recognised the wrong-doer and wanted him to change and be good. Sally particularly enjoyed displays of affection between Punch and Judy and any puppet antics such as clapping and waving which she would copy.

The child took the puppet baby away and rocked it. She did the same with Punch and showed signs of wanting to be in the play. Encouraged by her entreaties, the story was started again:

Everyone is asleep. (Sally was also pretending to be asleep, so I brought her in.) Punch is asleep, Sally is asleep, Judy is asleep. Who wakes up first? Sally pointed at Punch. She then put the baby down, brought in Judy and pushed Punch and Judy together for a kiss. (Sally clappped in appreciation.) She then gave the baby to Punch, pushed Judy away and fetched a policeman. (The play continued until Sally had had enough, which happened quite abruptly.)

She stood up, opened the sliding door of our room and then collapsed on to her knees once again and crawled away.

Sally used no speech, but she made noises, clapped, pointed or waved both hands at once.

Throughout the visit, on both days I worked with her, Sally responded to the puppets, following wherever they were being used. Her instincts were quite basic in relating to them, she showed fear of the crocodile, she was not attracted by the ghost, devil or the queen, but was interested in the less fantastic figures related more to her own experience.

These two examples demonstrate the use of puppets in different circumstances. One child had both an intellectual impairment

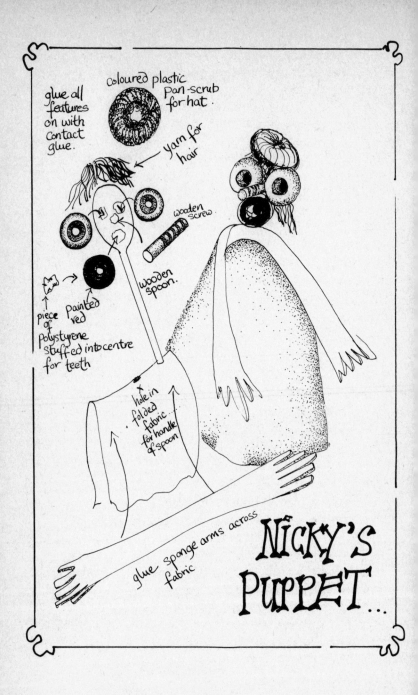

glue all features on with Contact glue.

Coloured plastic pan-scrub for hat.

yarn for hair

wooden screw.

↑ piece of Polystyrene stuffed into centre for teeth

painted red

wooden spoon.

X hole in folded fabric for handle of spoon

glue sponge arms across fabric

NICKY'S PUPPET...

and a physical handicap. She was in her classroom at school, and the puppet was used in a lesson which was not normally to include puppetry. The use of the art-form was to help the child override some of her problems in order to allow a learning experience to take place.

The second child seemed physically able but pretending not to be, and was much more severely retarded. The aim of the art-form in this instance was first to take the child out of her normal unstructured situation to get to know her better, and then to lead her into seeing her own circumstances at home more objectively through the puppets.

A more concentrated course in puppetry

The following example involves a child who had been diagnosed as autistic, and as far as could be judged appeared to be suffering a delay in language as a result of the autism. The sessions for this child stretched over four days, and concentrated on the child's ability to relate to others and his environment through new experience.

Although our approach to Nicky was to be informal we decided that there had to be a certain class structure. I was particularly interested in involving several twelve-year-old children with the problems of handicapped children. Before each class we planned which of them was going to work with Nicky and their approach to the task. These volunteers tried very hard to contribute to the sessions with Nicky but their lack of experience left them unable to anticipate his needs and the effects of his disability.

Nicky tended to gravitate towards me, perhaps because I was more confident of our relationship and perhaps because I was better able to offer alternatives when he lost concentration. The class had several aims:

1. To encourage Nicky to complete a job successfully, and to experience the pleasure of doing so;
2. To involve him physically with other children and to encourage him to play co-operatively;
3. To keep Nicky fruitfully occupied all day;

4. To give him the opportunity of more productive activity than he was normally used to.

The class started about 10 am. After our planning meeting, Nicky would arrive with his mother, who left him at the door. We allowed him to wander around the room looking at whatever interested him. The other children talked to him, and touching him was encouraged as a welcome—hugging, kissing or just a pat.

On the first day, we took Nicky shopping for the materials he needed to make his simple rod puppet (see page 100):

A wooden spoon
some wooden washers
a wooden screw
a tube of instant glue
a plastic pan-scrub.

Nicky paid for all these items, but the selection of materials and the handling of the money was carried out in a detached uncomprehending manner.

We went to a cafe and Nicky had a milk-shake. He was agitated about drinking it, but eventually did so with a great deal of encouragement. The whole outing was an experience for him. He was preoccupied with it all day and on occasions produced whole sentences, beaming all over his face. ''Milk shake, milk shake,'' and ''I had a milk shake'' and ''We went to a cafe.''

We started to make his rod puppet. He was made to select his own materials and to decide for himself on the location of features on the puppet's face. We did this by asking him to find his own nose for example, and then to find mine. In this way he increased his body awareness. By the end of the first day with us, using continuous questioning to guide the child's work, he had completed Mr Nosey. He had remembered, from summer school he had attended two months before, how to use contact glue, how to apply it and wait for it to dry before sticking the surfaces together. He was also still able to use scissors, but his hand-eye co-ordination was not good.

He had seen some of my own shows in the past and it was

not long before he started using a squeaky voice for his own puppet. With encouragement Nicky was able to:

Relate to his puppet;
Realise the puppet was for showing to others;
Respond to us wanting to see him use the puppet;
Use the puppet for communicating.

He also wanted me to join him and tell a story for Mr Nosey to act (Nicky thought up the name for the puppet himself).

When a piece of work was completed, Nicky was again allowed to wander around on his own. He habitually flapped one hand, so, to draw his attention to that obsessive movement, I would put a puppet into his hand.

On the second day Nicky was still interested in his story and when his concentration could be sustained he would happily tell it, using Mr Nosey. We allowed Nicky to play in whatever way he liked so long as it brought him into contact with the other children.

He spent much time going in and out of my Punch and Judy booth fiddling around with the zip. A game which gave him special pleasure was to jump up and peep over the playboard and say "hello". This was new for him, he was trying to create an impact on the rest of the class by showing off.

On the third day Nicky was preoccupied with a loose tooth. During the morning he was unable to concentrate so we went out into town. The afternoon brought no improvement in his attitude so I played a biting game with him. This led to growling and then the whole group became interested and talked about their dogs. From that game, Whiskey the dog puppet developed. The ideas came out of the group involvement, and they were realised by the same questioning method as we had used in making the other puppet:

"Where is his head? Where are his teeth? Where are your teeth? Does he have more teeth? Where is his back? Where is his tummy? Where is his tail?"

By the fourth day Nicky was showing more interest in the puppets of the other children, but no interest in making a puppet for himself.

CONTACT AND CONTROL OF THE PUPPETS ..

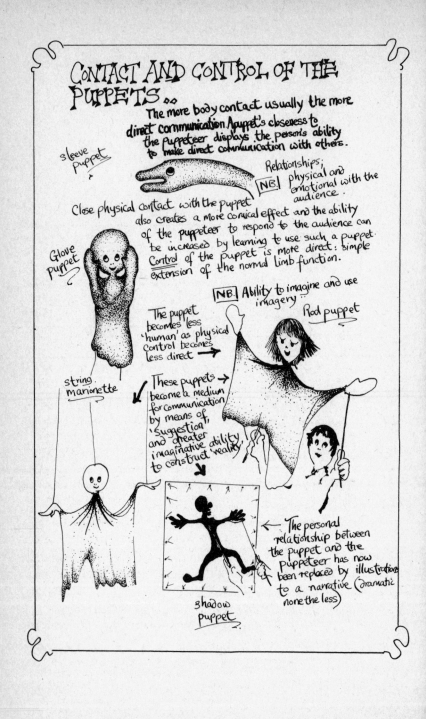

The more body contact usually the more direct communication. A puppet's closeness to the puppeteer displays the person's ability to make direct communication with others.

Sleeve puppet

NB. Relationships; physical and emotional with the audience.

Close physical contact with the puppet also creates a more comical effect and the ability of the puppeteer to respond to the audience can be increased by learning to use such a puppet. Control of the puppet is more direct: simple extension of the normal limb function.

Glove puppet

NB. Ability to imagine and use imagery.

Rod puppet

The puppet becomes less 'human' as physical control becomes less direct →

These puppets → become a medium for communication by means of 'suggestion' and greater imaginative ability to construct 'reality'.

String marionette

← The personal relationship between the puppet and the puppeteer has now been replaced by illustration to a narrative (dramatic none the less)

shadow puppet

Nicky's family were enthusiastic about the improvement they saw in him during the week. They said he was no longer a shadow but a real "presence".

Nicky became lively, more adventurous and prepared to relate to the other people. Some simple ideas that he had he was able to realise through art and he experienced pride in his achievement.

In this last section we have been looking at the use of the puppet in quite unusual circumstances. The puppets have not been used in typical "show" situations but more or less one-to-one with a therapist or teacher, a puppet and a child. The puppet has been used as a means towards solving another problem. The subject in each case was using his ability to animate an inanimate object and was therefore introducing a whole new element into the normal classroom or therapy situation.

We shall now proceed to examining puppetry in drama: as an art-form "for its own sake".

The same assessment criteria will be used as before—they are relevant throughout work with puppets.

It will be useful at this stage to glance at the illustration on page 104, showing the different aspects of body contact between puppet and puppeteer. If the person to use the puppets has any behaviour problems, or has difficulty in relating to other people, then it is better to start off with a less intimate form of puppet communication, with the shadow puppets—either screen or overhead projector. The goal would then be eventually to be able to use the close body contact puppets, sleeve and glove.

PART THREE

Dramatic Structure

What is drama?
Questions for the teacher
Exercises in play-making
a) Hand puppets with alternative plots and a note on drama and play
b) Shadow puppets

Dramatic Structure

What is drama?

DRAMA is the action resulting from ideas in opposition. Such action is presented through the creative means available to the person.

Our view of reality is represented in drama in the following four ways:

Movement	expressed artistically through: mime, dance, action (within the role)
Vocalisation	expressed artistically through: speech, song
Sound	expressed artistically through: music, sound effects
Ideas	expressed artistically through: the role character

These points are very much simplified. They will, however, help to present the beginning of structured drama for the less able. By using the above outline, you will be providing the framework to enable a handicapped person to express himself more fully.

Identification of the role

A character is identified by the way he looks and the way he acts. The handicapped artist may however need extra reinforcement of the character, and this may be done *visually* by use of make-up, masks or puppets: and *aurally* by use of special sound effects, music and song which are appropriate to the character. In many cases it is important to use as many types of reinforcement as possible. Clear identification of the character and the part he plays in relation to other characters is vital to the puppeteer's ability to take control of the situation: to become master, in other words.

WHAT IS DRAMA ?

opposing ideas in action

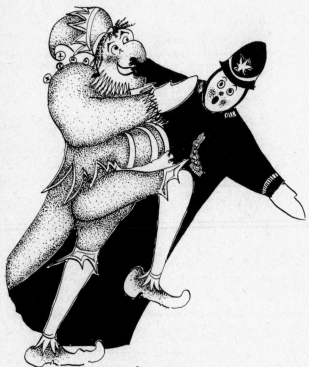

Punch (we know → meets Policeman → something
him by the way he   (we know him by   happens.
looks, acts, moves,   the way he looks   What ?
speaks)   acts, moves, speaks

The characters must be consistent with their make-up .

WHAT IS DRAMA?

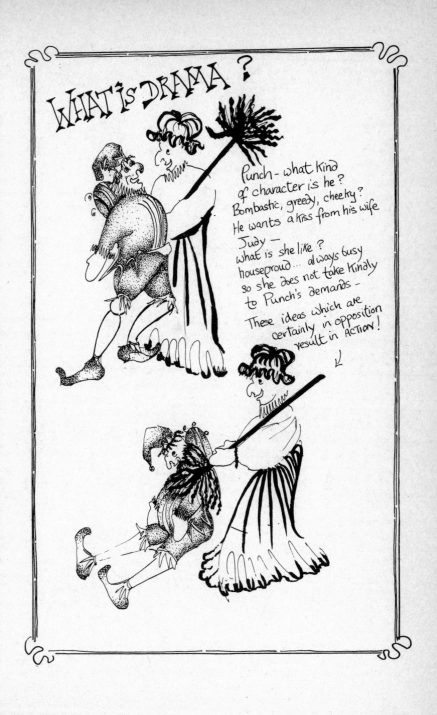

Punch – what kind of character is he?
Bombastic, greedy, cheeky?
He wants a kiss from his wife

Judy –
what is she like?
houseproud... always busy
so she does not take kindly
to Punch's demands –

These ideas which are
certainly in opposition
result in ACTION!

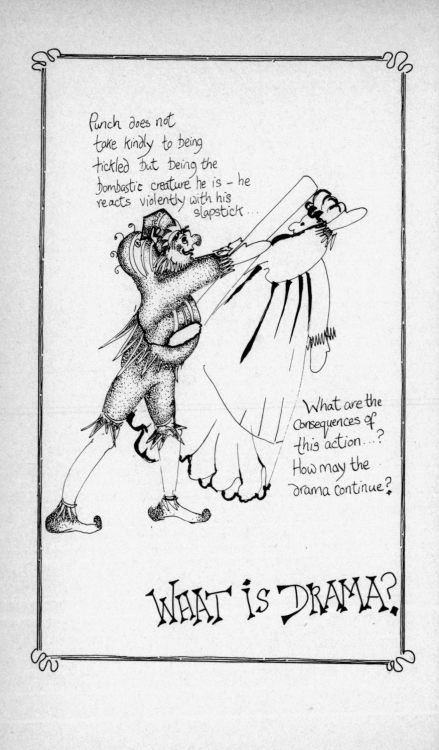

You will notice that I use a great deal of colour and costume. I have chosen to use that kind of imagery. It is my signature, so to speak, but I find that clearly defined characters, richly imaginative in conception, are important to stimulate others to use the puppets.

Once the character is established and clearly reinforced as described, the opportunity exists for drama to develop. The most direct way for this to happen is between two characters, both easily identifiable. A dramatic conflict can be expressed with one person only, perhaps struggling with a problem inside himself and expressing his problem as an argument with himself through the four dramatic means of expression we have described. Or on the other hand the dramatic conflict can be between various groups of characters, each holding to a particular ideology. But in order to develop drama with a person who is mentally handicapped it is best at first to simplify by limiting action to two characters.

The pace of the action
The play or scene may be governed by the rhythmic beating of musical instruments or other sound effects. The rhythmic pattern may at the same time be used to reinforce the developing picture of the character in the mind of the artist. If we return to our definition of drama as the action arising from contrasted ideas, then the most easily identified situations will be those around opposing characters: good/bad, comic/sad, clever/stupid.

Suppose that we start with a discussion among students. We may conclude that "bad" characters are aggressive, so we accompany them with heavy rhythmic music. The "good" characters are then by contrast kept free of a regular pattern, and lighter toned music is used. Then we begin to improvise with puppets, each improvisation lasting only a few minutes, since a mentally handicapped person may have difficulty in sustaining a scene for long. An actual performance can be made up of a combination of scenes, consisting of action between different pairs of characters—which is the way the traditional Punch and Judy show is constructed. The teacher should be prepared to take the main part, with the other performers taking one puppet and one piece of action each.

Characters should be clearly identifiable;
Situations should be clearly established;
Scenes should be brief;
Music can be used to dictate the rhythm of the action, and to reinforce character.

The aim of using such a strict structure for the drama is to provide a safe framework in which the person is free to develop artistically. Remember that it is easy to steer a person through a process but much more difficult to encourage her to think for herself. Art is sometimes thought to mean total freedom of self-expression—"letting it all go", "letting it all hang out!" But though this may be a movement in art, I do not see it as allowing real freedom in creativity at all. The creative process is a critical process, and the framework is the medium for expression. A person who is mentally handicapped needs to be encouraged to use an objective art-form in which the symbols are easily recognisable so that a measure of communication is easily maintained. Puppetry is an opportunity to *objectify* emotions in the puppet and act them out in a dramatic situation. Ideas are expressed *through* the puppet.

Questions for the teacher

Are ideas being expressed clearly through the puppet? Are those ideas appropriate to the character? Could other source material be used—e.g. stories, pictures, film—to provide additional information about the character?

Can you provide additional reinforcement in the way of a song or catch-phrase to help the person performing the puppet to know who he is in the role? Is the person in physical control of the puppet—is he *master*?

Performing Boris the Bad in subnormality hospitals

We spent three days away—one day at each of a group of three subnormality hospitals. The time was arranged in this way: each morning was spent running workshops, to which were sent groups of eight to ten residents; we also went to wards whose residents were not going to be able to come to see the show later on; and in the afternoons we put on performances of *Boris the Bad* for staff and residents.

The aim of the workshops was to prepare the residents for the main performance. Some of the people were very severely handicapped, all were long institutionalised and none had any previous experience of the kind we were to offer.

The puppets were introduced one by one to each person. Some residents were expected to hold a puppet and use it in response to questions from the puppeteer, or to actions by another puppet. Other people worked with the assistant, a musician, trying out simple instruments: drum, cymbals, tambourine, recorder.

Each character was a caricature type: Bad Boris, Good Peter, Fat King, Nondescript Queen, Girly girl, Feathery bird, Fag Ash Lil.

Each character had his own distinctive features, a song or sound to accompany him, and characteristic movement. No more than two characters were used at a time and their entrances and exits were emphasised by the use of their own song, catch-phrases and special movements. Each character was thus identified by the way he looked and the way he acted. Throughout the plot scenes of similar content were repeated. There was also much repetition of dialogue and action within scenes.

The result was that most of the people attending the sessions were able to concentrate for the whole half to three quarter-hour period. Each puppet was recognised, and the actors soon achieved good co-ordination between puppets and music. Some of the more able were beginning to anticipate the action on the basis of their understanding of the characters.

But what was most interesting from the performer's point of view was the way in which this way of working together actually changed the play. When something in the original plot was obviously not getting through to the mentally handi-capped improvisers, ideas were re-worked and re-worked until they could be presented in a way acceptable to the group. The Queen character had to be dropped from the show—her characterisation was simply not clear enough, so she was hard to include in any improvisation. Eventually Fag

CHARACTER

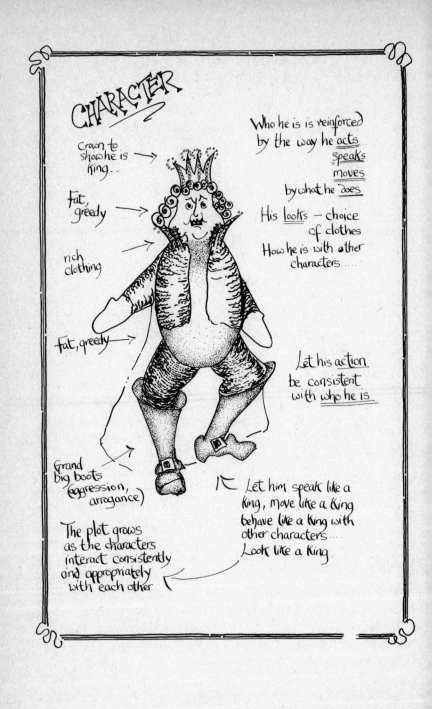

Crown to show he is King...

Fat, greedy

rich clothing

Fat, greedy

Grand big boots (aggression, arrogance)

The plot grows as the characters interact consistently and appropriately with each other

Who he is is reinforced by the way he acts
speaks
moves
by what he does
His looks — choice of clothes
How he is with other characters......

Let his action be consistent with who he is

Let him speak like a King, move like a King behave like a King with other characters....
Look like a King.

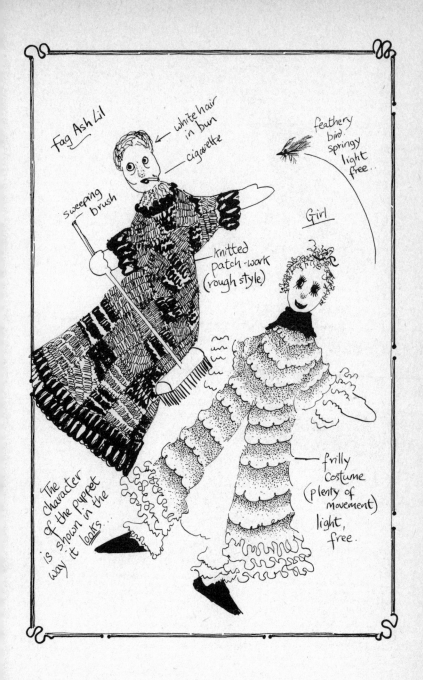

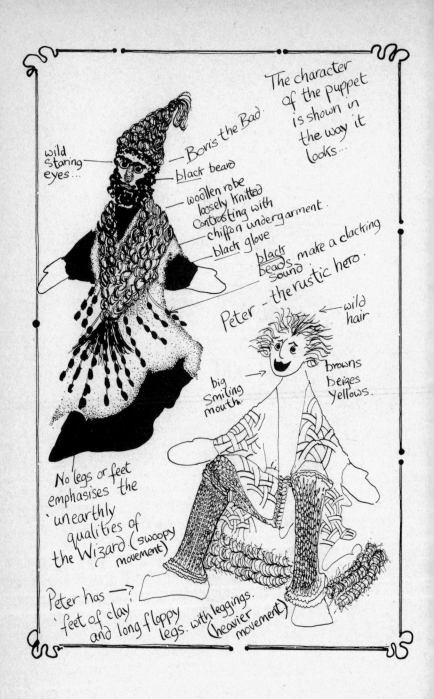

wild
staring
eyes...

—Boris the Bad.

black beard

woollen robe
loosely knitted
contrasting with
chiffon undergarment.

black glove

black beads make a clacking sound

The character of the puppet is shown in the way it looks...

Peter - the rustic hero.

wild hair

browns
beiges
yellows.

big smiling mouth.

No legs or feet emphasises the 'unearthly' qualities of the Wizard (swoopy movement)

Peter has —>
'feet of clay' and long floppy legs. with leggings. (heavier movement)

Ash Lil became the King's mother, as a mother-child relationship was easy for the people to understand. For a while Fag Ash Lil was Peter's mother, but Peter, as the hero, became submerged in too many relationships when he had both mother and girl-friend. There was another character for a short time — Ivan the 'Orrible, a mercenary — but he caused complications because he was another bad character and represented a sub-plot which spoilt the flow of the main plot. The response was much clearer when Boris reigned supreme as the one and only and worst baddie of the lot!

What was happening was that the show was literally growing out of the creative minds of these very severely handicapped and thoroughly institutionalised adults. Accordingly, on the second day I and the assistant completely reset the show at lunchtime in time for the afternoon performance, entirely according to the ideas expressed by the groups during that morning.

The responses to the puppets varied among the different hospitals. The men in the all-male ward were less able to comprehend and less responsive than the women in the all-female ward, but best of all was the mixed hospital, where the residents were much more able to understand the relationships between the puppets of opposite sex: boy-friend/girl-friend, mother/son, bad man/good girl. If the plot is to grow out of these relationships, an inability to understand them obviously makes further progress difficult.

Response to the professional puppets was also markedly different from that to the home-made dolls they had worked with in a previous year. And we had no doubt that the workshop groups had had a direct bearing on the success of the main show: the repetition and improvisation helped those who were the most disabled to respond more intelligently to the drama, and the slightly more able in effect became helpers.

Let us look again at our checklist (page 24), and apply it to this experiment:

1. Did the people in the groups relate to the puppets? Yes, most people tried to react in a way appropriate (with

encouragement from puppeteer) to all the puppets with very clearly defined characters.

2. Did they recognise that puppets were for showing to people? Some individuals were afraid to put their hands inside the puppets but they were prepared to "perform" holding the puppets, like ordinary dolls, with their hands safely where they could see them!

3. Did they rise to expectations? Usually the groups responded to my demands to perform to me. It was hard work sometimes, however, except in the cases of those who were deaf and mute, who all happened to be very lively and expressive. Unfortunately none of them used any kind of signing.

4. Did the above experiment make use of the puppets to extend the social repertoire of the group members? In many cases there were genuine and intelligent efforts to communicate *through* the puppet. Personal feelings were expressed about the issues of the plot, and the moral choices made by the puppets were understood (this came through in the main show later on each day).

5. In what ways did each person "act" appropriately with the puppet? The ability to role play emerged as a person "became" the character and was able to act in character consistently. Boris for instance was bad, and acted bad every time he came on.

6. How did the performers show sensitivity to the audience? In the workshops there was no large audience to bring out a response, but each group was much guided by *my* response to them, and my response gave direction and enabled them to build on the next action.

I have told this story in detail to show how clearly identifiable characters and situations help the creative process of drama to develop. Characters *must* be convincing and *must* convey ideas—opposing ideas then spark off the dramatic situation, and the plot grows. Ideas are implicit in the look of the character, which stimulates the action.

Exercises in play-making

What is the next step? We shall now look again at puppetry as a performance art. At this point many people begin to question how they can justify puppetry with those who are handicapped. Puppets have indeed been used with some success to help people overcome specific problems, but is there a case for going further? Should we not be spending our time with mentally handicapped people towards more practical ends? Remember, I am discussing this from the point of view of a professional artist. I don't practise my art for any other reason than for its own sake. Does a policeman or doctor have to justify what he does? Nevertheless, I got to the stage where I felt I had to justify myself and my work and apologise for my sense of achievement and enjoyment. Similarly, a teacher who had been on one of my courses, who had had a frame built and even started to make a collection of puppets, also panicked—how could she possibly justify puppetry for its own sake? She felt she ought to be doing something *educational*, and hers and my enjoyment in what we were doing was incompatible with that!

Plain and simply then, a person being creative needs in his daily experience adequate opportunity to express himself fully. Art provides a means of self-expression and in that provision is healing: the means of reconciling a person to himself and to the world around him. What could be more useful and practical to a handicapped person?

(a) Hand puppets

Performance can thus be enjoyed simply for what it is. The following work is to introduce puppetry as an art-form, with any therapeutic value implicit rather than explicit.

Excercise 1

At a table. This has been chosen for a number of reasons:

  1. The table provides a barrier between the therapist and the patient;
  2. It is somewhere to rest your arms;

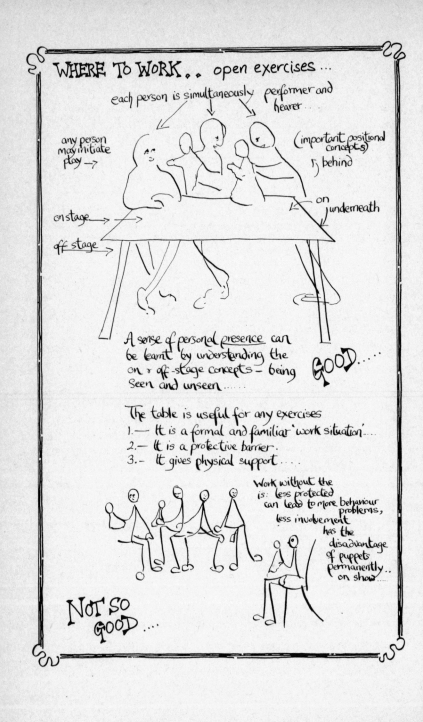

WHERE TO WORK.. open exercises...

each person is simultaneously performer and hearer...

any person may initiate play →

(important positional concepts)

↳ behind

on

underneath

on stage →

off stage →

A sense of personal presence can be learnt by understanding the on & off-stage concepts — being seen and unseen.......

GOOD.....

The table is useful for any exercises
1.— It is a formal and familiar 'work situation'....
2.— It is a protective barrier.
3.— It gives physical support....

Work without the is: less protected can lead to more behaviour problems, less involvement has the disadvantage of puppets permanently on show.....

NOT SO GOOD....

3. It gives dimension to the activity: underneath, on top, behind, in front. This could for instance be important for language work;

4. The table provides formality. It is known as a place where one eats, works, plays some games. It is a place of activity.

Ways of working:

1. Encourage the members of the group to keep a good sitting position. Ask them to stand up and sit down a number of times to check on their balance. (Make a game out of this)

2. Ask who would like to hold the puppets. Promise each person a turn.

3. Introduce a puppet, such as the King. Using a character voice to ask the group some questions:

Do you like my clothes?

What colour is my jacket?

Where is my crown? I've lost my crown!

Where are my boots? I've lost my boots!

The King has forgotten what he looks like and this problem with himself presents us with a dramatic problem: Can he find his boots without help from the group? Will they or won't they help him?

What have I got for breakfast?

In preparation for this last question, have ready cut-out colour photographs (from magazines) of breakfast foods, glued on to paper plates.

4. Call the cooks! What have *you* brought me for breakfast? (Allow each person to say or show what they have brought the King for breakfast.)

The purpose of this activity is to encourage involvement between the group members and the puppet. As the puppeteer you must also be very convincing, and relate well to the puppet. Make him move around and greet each member of the group—YOU MUST PERFORM. You are encouraging the members to act playfully with the puppet. Be prepared to laugh and to show that you are enjoying yourself.

The session could easily end there.

You should have established the table-top as the playing area, stage or playboard. Make a great deal of this. Remember that you are introducing puppetry as an art-form and not as random play. What happened during the improvisation? Did you allow people to lie across the table, put their heads down, or go to sleep? The special area for performance should be demonstrated by the effective use of the puppet upon it. If the space becomes identified with the puppet characters, you will find fewer attempts to sprawl on it! You could stick down some coloured paper or covering to make the playing area more distinctive. A loose cloth is not such a good idea as it muffles the sounds of the puppets' feet and can easily slide off.

The short session is necessary to establish the immediate reactions of the group. At first keep in the group only the most responsive people. As you work on their positive reactions, you will gradually be building a group who will not only be able to work the puppets but will also encourage you if you are not very experienced as a performer. If *all* members of the selected group are responding to the puppet (by gesture or by verbal communication), you will be ready to move on to another session immediately. The next session will involve your students in handling puppets. You will need a chef-type puppet (page 129).

Exercise 2

1. You may repeat the wording of the previous session, but at some point introduce the new puppets to one person at a time. Direct all instructions to the puppets and not to the puppeteers. Your objective in this session should be to encourage the group members to relate to their own puppets by interaction with the principal puppet that you are handling—the King. The King should be in character all the time. Try to avoid coming out of character, so speak *through* the puppet even if you are not actually using scripted dialogue. If you need to speak as yourself, allow the puppet to excuse himself, take him out of sight, or simply take your hand out and lay the puppet on the playboard.

2. Have only one character working with the main character at a time (no more than two puppets appearing at one time).
3. Once again the session should be kept brief, just a few minutes.
4. You should at the end of this session have established in the minds of the group the idea that when worked the puppet "comes alive", and when not being worked the puppet is just a doll. Keep on reminding the students of this "the doll is just a doll—when I have my hand inside I make the puppet come alive!" Demonstrate the contrast. That each person has control of the puppet and that the puppet is going to do as she tells it, is also important for each person to know. These are aspects of animation vital to understand.
5. Each person must also understand the moments of non-involvement. When she is not working her puppet, it lies at rest, and then the puppeteer becomes audience for the others at the table. This does not involve changing places but simply a change of attitude. The principal puppet can lead each puppeteer and puppet as they come to the end of their few seconds of performance by telling the puppeteer to lay down the puppet and to watch what is going on.
6. It is important that each person becomes emotionally "disengaged" from the action in order to make an intelligent and objective appraisal of each part of the improvisation. This is done by establishing a routine for the removal of each puppet.

The next session takes the group into the essence of drama: action resulting from ideas in opposition. You will still be leading the group with the principal character, but now all the other group members should have puppets. Select puppets which are clearly characterised by their appearance.

The above methodical approach has been adopted not simply to be able to measure visible responses, but to make an intellectual appreciation possible for the less able members of the group. The sessions described allow for intellectual, critical and emotional growth through art. The success of this approach will be evident as time goes on and individuals make choices for themselves, becoming more involved in puppetry in different ways. Expressing himself through the art of puppetry, each person—handicapped or not—will be making decisions at the moment of every artistic move, *not* at the completion of the activity. But it takes work to reach that moment of pure inspiration.

With people who are extremely institutionalised, it is important to be ready for over-reactions to the puppets. Responses can be unpredictable especially where the ability to reason is limited. So if you are going to work with groups of mentally handicapped people you will need to have some experience as a performer, as well as be familiar with people who are disabled in this way. Although a violin teacher may not have actually made his own violin, if he intends to teach others to play he must be able to play himself. Similarly, the teacher must know how to perform with puppets. Experience as a performer also leaves one sensitive to the whole range of emotional response, both in the audience and in the puppeteer. Here the *professional artist* has much to contribute to the treatment of handicapped people. It is also more realistic to use puppets in therapy *after* patients have been exposed to puppetry as art in performance.

I remember once travelling a very long way to speak as a guest at a conference. I had my "thesis" with me and my experimental examples (puppets) packed into a very full suitcase. As a performer I was feeling very insecure in the presence of medical people. They used terms for people and problems that I had never heard before. I spent a miserable lunchtime wishing I had read all the right books and had gone to medical lectures instead of spending all those hours drawing naked statues in the Victoria and Albert Museum. As I began to speak I felt more and more embarrassed: because I had a suitcase full of puppets, because people would be able to see I was on the wrong track, because all these experts were talkers and no one could disprove *words*. And what was even worse, I could see so many newspapers—NO ONE WAS LISTENING.' Lecturers may be used to that, but to a peformer it is a nightmare! I talked simply about the opportunities I had had to work alongside doctors and therapists, about the designing of puppets for special use and I referred warmly to my "friends", Simon, Tubby, Ted and the others, when I produced one after another out of the case. Gradually newspapers were lowered, a television team was alerted and people started to bristle with questions—where could they get puppets like those? I also explained that I had never attempted to assess the success or failure of my own work with handicapped people, but left this to those more qualified to do so, if I was working as part of a specialist team.

I came away from that conference confirmed in my belief that the performing artist has a part to play in the treatment of any handicapped person.

Art and play

It is important to distinguish between art and play. One has only to glance at the play of children to be immediately impressed by the randomness of their activity, in time and space and content. The intensity changes, the alterations in mood are remarkable. Each play has its own structure by a sort of mutual agreement, but this too may change at any moment to be replaced or adapted. From concentration on the sensual enjoyment of materials in physical play, concept formation progresses the child into ideological play, much of which is dramatic. Chases are early games of this type, all the children taking the same part, and later on, as moral values are formed and expressed, different children act more and more individually, taking different parts as principal protagonists emerge. Lone play evolves into "art" quite early as the child brings you things he has made or takes you along to see what he has done. But dramatic play remains play for much longer, and until the child is much older the same fantasy, perhaps even the same game, continues perhaps for hours, weeks, months. If the child uses puppets, the same ideas are sometimes repeated for weeks at a time. Puppets *confine* dramatic play, so that it remains a more private activity for the child. Gradually, as the ideas of the child mature, play is *replaced* by art and the drama becomes the medium for the conscious communication of ideas to others. Although one could possibly say that art follows play in some kind of developmental sequence, the two are certainly not one and the same. The young performer may call more and more for others to share—but as *audience*, not to participate except in very very minor roles under his direction.

If play opens the eyes of the child to all her creative potential, then one can understand the deprivation of the child who is unable to play for any reason. For such people, art can to some extent replace what is missing through lack of the early experience of play. Play on the other hand cannot be reintroduced as the spontaneous random activity it is by definition. For handicapped people who are unable to play, art must offer the experience for growth instead. Play is its own reward and gratifies needs immediately. The immediacy of a performing art like puppetry can serve in a similar way.

Exercise 3

Follow the same method as before, introducing the puppets one at a time, then encouraging someone to play each of the subsidiary parts, but playing the main part yourself. Try some of these plots to act with a small group (pages 130–133).

A character is sweeping the floor, singing a sweeping song. Every time she stops and turns her back a little mouse creeps on with more rubbish—just when she thinks she has finished. At first she thinks she has forgotten the rubbish, then she gets suspicious, then she hides and watches what is happening, then she rushes out and chases the mouse away.

A snappy crocodile is lying in HIS river. On one side of the river a little girl is stranded, fast asleep. On the other side of the river are three friends, one with a big stick, the other with a net and the third with nothing at all. One at a time they try to get to the other side, but each time the crocodile beats them back by stealing first the stick and then the net. The man who has nothing says he will have a go, the others laugh because he has no weapon at all. He says he believes in magic—so he prays for a spell and to the surprise of the others his legs grow and grow and grow until he is tall enough to step over the river and rescue the girl, and the crocodile can do nothing about it.

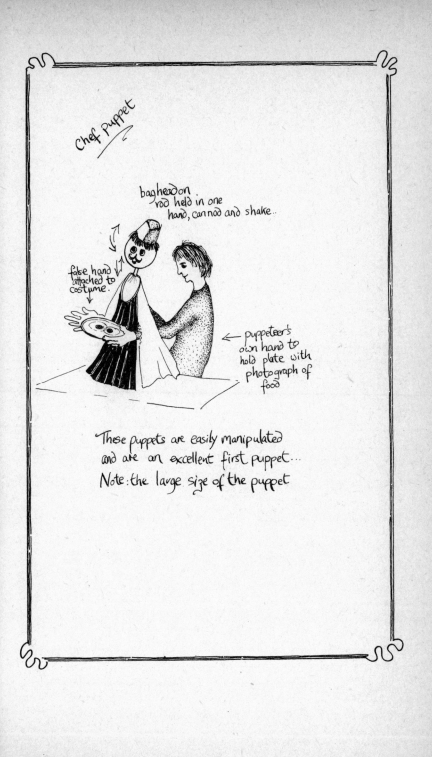

Chef Puppet

bag head on rod held in one hand, can nod and shake..

false hand attached to costume.

← puppeteer's own hand to hold plate with photograph of food

These puppets are easily manipulated
and are an excellent first puppet...
Note: the large size of the puppet

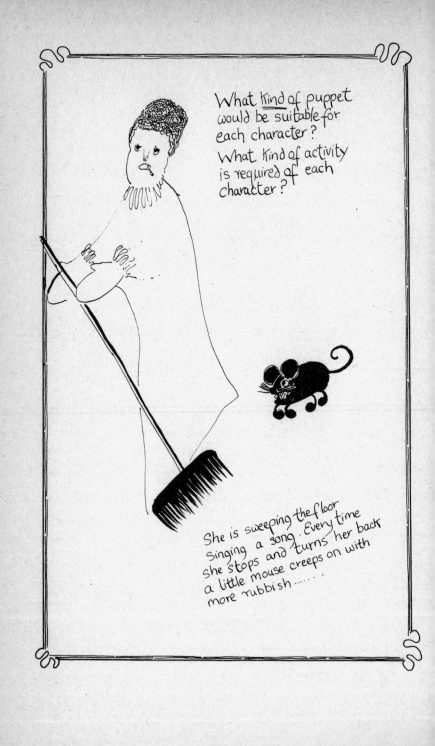

What kind of puppet would be suitable for each character?

What kind of activity is required of each character?

She is sweeping the floor singing a song. Every time she stops and turns her back a little mouse creeps on with more rubbish........

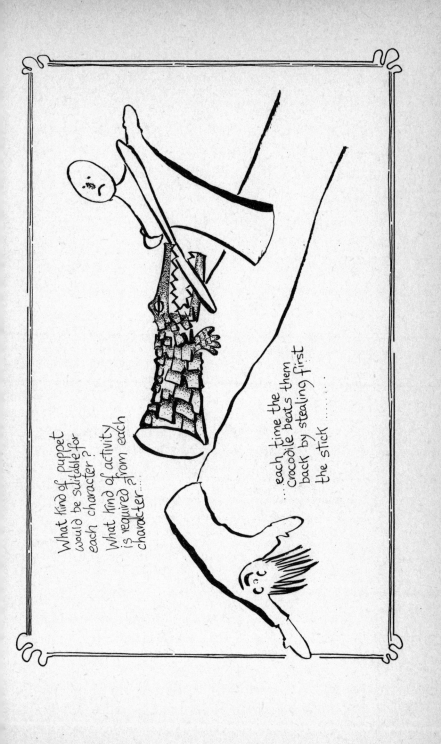

What kind of puppet would be suitable for each character?

What kind of activity is required from each character......

...each time the crocodile beats them back by stealing first the stick ....

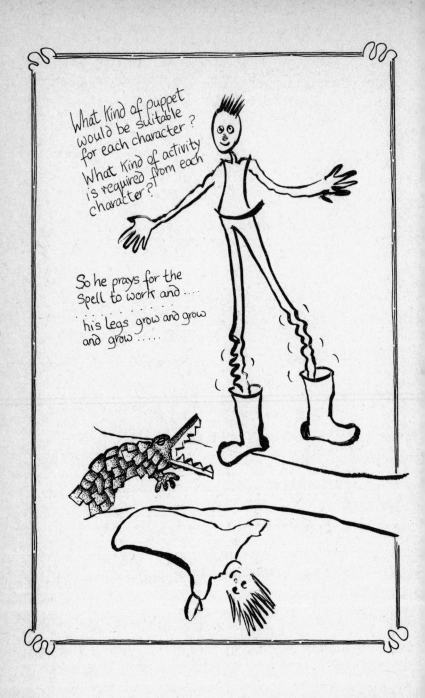

What kind of puppets
would be suitable for
each character?

What kind of activity
is required of each
character?

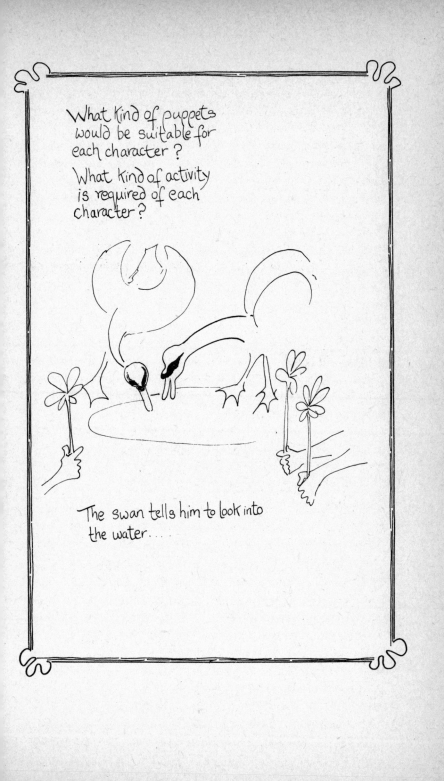

The swan tells him to look into
the water.....

Once there was an ugly duckling. His brothers and sisters one by one chase him away by laughing at him and pecking him. He goes away, and falls asleep. The snow comes and falls on him. The flowers come up. Some swans come and they find him and ask him why he is hiding—because he is so ugly and the other ducks laugh at him. The swan tells him to look into the water—and then he sees he has changed into a lovely swan himself.

With the exception of the long-legs story, these can be performed at the table booth after they have been prepared at the flat table. Always encourage interested people to watch the little performances. Of course your groups are part audience and part performers at all times as only two puppets ever appear at once.

(b) Shadow puppets

Table work is excellent as a start to glove, sleeve and rod puppetry, but it is not suitable for shadow puppets, as the latter need their own set up.

The best way to approach shadow puppetry is by means of a show of your own. It is a good idea to have helper(s) in the audience as you will not actually be able to see what they are seeing from the other side of the screen. Shadow puppets are ideal for story-telling, and have proved extremely successful with mentally handicapped people.

Exercise 4

1. First perform a simple story with more than one character, and invite members of the group one by one to join you behind the screen to take over the working of the puppets.

2. Then give each member of the group a puppet. Work in pairs, one showing the other the puppet and then changing roles. At the end of this session each person should be able to work her own puppet, to show signs of being able to recognise the puppet both on and off the screen, and to place her puppet on the appropriate part of the screen: top, bottom, top middle, bottom middle, side etc. It might be

WHERE TO WORK.. concealed exercises...

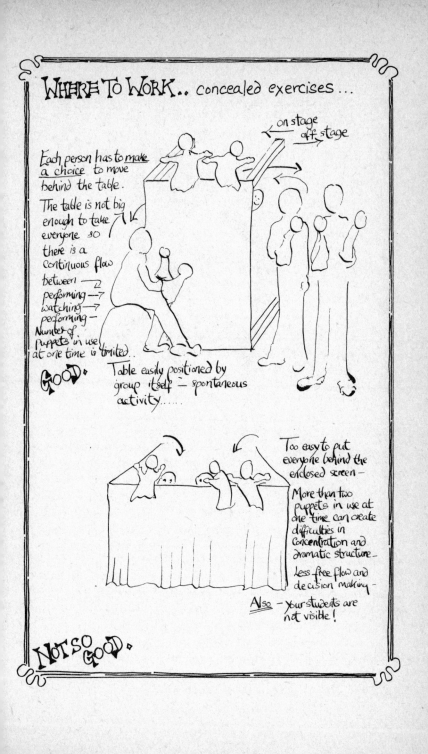

on stage
off stage

Each person has to make a choice to move behind the table.

The table is not big enough to take everyone so there is a continuous flow between
performing →
watching →
performing —

Number of puppets in use at one time is limited..

GOOD.

Table easily positioned by group itself — spontaneous activity......

Too easy to put everyone behind the enclosed screen —

More than two puppets in use at one time can create difficulties in concentration and dramatic structure—

Less free flow and decision making —

Also — your students are not visible!

NOT SO GOOD.

WHERE TO WORK ... the shadow screen.....

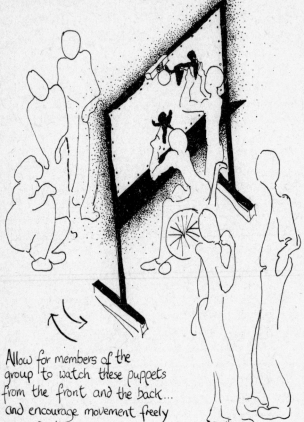

Allow for members of the
group to watch these puppets
from the front and the back...
and encourage movement freely
around the screen...

The screen is to become an exciting and special place
in the same way as the table-booth and the table-top...

necessary to spend a few days at this stage, but you can find other ways of teaching the same lesson by varying your story. When the whole group has achieved this it will be time to move on to the next stage.

Here is a story suitable for this early work.

Once upon a time there lived a mouse in the corner of the screen. It was his screen. He decided to go for a walk all around the screen because it was his screen. Off he goes. Across the bottom of the screen into the other corner. Up the side to the top corner. Across the top. Into the other corner. And down, down the side. "Oh! What's that in the middle of my screen?" squeaked the mouse. "What is it? Oh no, it's a cat!" The mouse had to think hard. It was his screen, wasn't it? He had to get rid of the cat. Very, very slowly the mouse crept back up to the corner. Very, very slowly he crept to the top of the screen and he stopped in the middle. Then with a great big EEK he dropped right down on to the cat. "Miaaaow" went the cat and ran away. The mouse went back into the corner of his screen and curled up and went to sleep. It was HIS screen.

It is clear exactly what the objective is in using the story: notice the references to the positions on the screen, the easily recognisable puppets, the variation in the speed of action and the surprise at the end. You can imagine your own variations on the same story.

How can you now develop the work in following sessions? Give others the cat and mouse, for a start. What else would be suitable? Introduce a bird and a piece of cheese.

Exercise 5
The bird is flying around in the sky. There he is right at the top of the screen—backwards and forwards backwards and forwards and upside down. The bird has some cheese in his mouth for tea. The cat has seen the bird. She dashes out to get him. He flies away and drops the cheese. The cat has gone. The bird has gone. Look who's coming? Who is it?

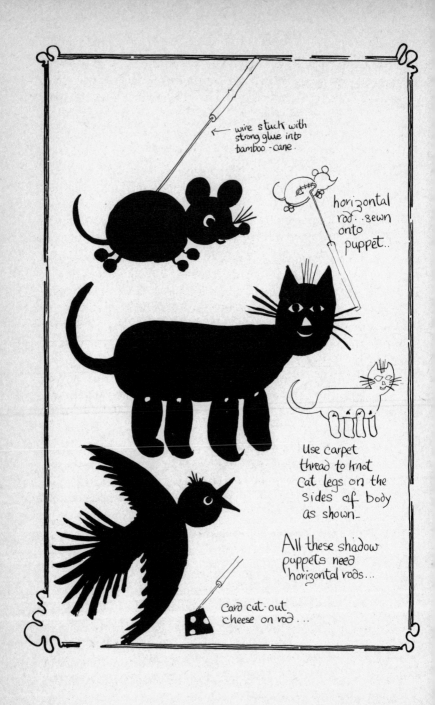

wire stuck with strong glue into bamboo-cane.

horizontal rod..sewn onto puppet..

Use carpet thread to knot cat legs on the sides of body as shown.

All these shadow puppets need horizontal rods...

Card cut-out cheese on rod...

The mouse? The mouse has seen the cheese. He runs up and gets it. The mouse is having the cheese for tea now. And he nibbles it and nibbles it until it is all gone.

Now in the story we have the free movement of the bird across the screen, unconnected to any base—a new dimension. Contrast the swooping of the bird with the quick dash of the cat and then the scurrying movement of the mouse.

This is all you need for a first show. Two people could perform the whole sequence on their own. Select who is going to be audience first and then who wants to perform. Take turns—helpers as well.

There is one more element of shadow puppetry still to be introduced, and that is a workable hinged joint. See instructions page 140–141.

Exercise 6

One day a great big tom-cat came to live near the screen. He crept up on the bird one day . . . slowly . . . slowly and then pounced, pounced on to him and tossed the poor little bird into the air with his nose and swallowed him. Then he crept up to where the little mouse was sleeping and pounced on him and swallowed him too . . . and he was still hungry. He saw the lump of cheese, he started to eat that too. But the hungry tiger came in. He crept up to the tom-cat and with one gulp swallowed the cat whole.

At one of the hospital schools we visited the audience was asked if they would like to come out and have a turn with the shadow puppets. A number of the children and young people did so. They were each given a puppet. They all saw how the light worked and they were interested in the shadows cast by their own hands. I invented a story to link up the puppets selected by the group. Behind the screen the volunteers had to listen for their cues and move to follow a simple narration. There was a teacher behind the screen to help them.

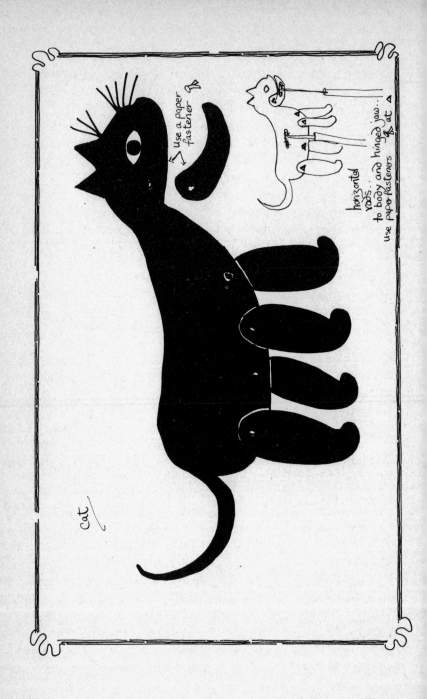

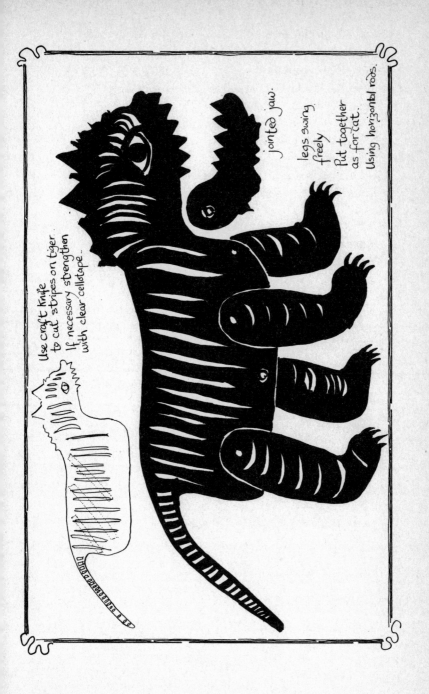

Use craft knife
to cut stripes on tiger.
If necessary strengthen
with clear cellotape.

jointed jaw.

legs swing
freely

Put together
as for cat.

Using horizontal rods.

Once upon a time there was a Mighty Mouse.
(The puppet appears and at the same time the corresponding
sound is made by a member of the audience)
He lived on the screen with:
a lady (puppet appears to sound of tambourine)
a little boy (penny whistle sound)
a little girl (triangle sound).

One day a nasty old ogre carrying a big stick came
stamping in (audience stamp feet). He frightened the people
away.

But in came Mighty Mouse and *he* frightened the ogre so
much that he ran away too. And the mouse called the people
back and they all danced.

The above was used as a game to link the audience with the
performers. Some increasingly complicated stories were
developed, and the excitement was gripping as they all waited
to hear their cues. The shadow puppets were simply
manipulated and extremely effective, accessible even for the
profoundly handicapped. I remember one boy in particular
came around the back of the screen. I gave him a puppet, and
he took it, but kept jerking his head back towards the wall
behind him. He continued doing this, becoming more and
more agitated, until I noticed that he was indicating a record
player high up on the top of a trolley. One of the nurses put on
a record, the boy turned to the screen and made his puppet
dance!

PART FOUR

Puppets as Special Aids
Machinery, music and vocal language
Puppets in speech therapy
Special problems
Multiply handicapped people
Social training
When puppets are not popular

Puppets as Special Aids

Machinery, music and vocal language

PUPPETRY as an art-form has been going on for thousands of years—we can see it illustrated in old paintings and even in the decorations on ancient pottery. In essence it has changed very little, for the animation aspects of the art must always remain the same. But there are some modern inventions helpful to teachers and therapists working with the handicapped. Modern materials and glues we have already examined, but what about machinery?

It is always surprising to see the amount of technical equipment available in an ordinary home. Most of us *do* live in an electronic age—yet many craft activities seem to have been permanently sewn, knitted or woven into a cottage industry era.

I remember working with a group of children—mixed ages with various problems—and deciding for the first time to use an overhead projector. A five-year-old however became most distressed and the whole class was disrupted. I eventually managed to gather from him that he was frightened by the noise of the projector. Noise? I listened. Sure enough, there was a noise, the noise of the fan. "Oh—you don't need to be afraid of that! Inside the box there's a fan going round and round and round keeping the engine cool—look . . ." and before I had a chance to continue there were nine pairs of enquiring eyes peering through the grille to see inside the machine better. I explained in a very amateur way about how the projector works to a very attentive group. I was greatly surprised. I don't know how much the children learnt, but I learnt that as an artist working *today* in the twentieth century I had to begin to use modern technology creatively.

Suggestions:
  1. Make tape recordings of simple conversations, and co-

ordinate these with puppets being worked by the original speakers. *Or* get the speakers to co-ordinate their tapes with the puppets—learning which buttons to press, and when.

2. Make recordings of different effects, such as water, cars, people singing, music, doors opening and closing, and then co-ordinate those to the action.

3. Use the overhead projector to project colour or scenery on to the main shadow screen, or use more than one projector to mix up different images. Fix dimmer switches on to the lights to allow for different effects. Teach the group members to fade lights gently, and to change colours and effects. (Make sure all electrical equipment is safe.)

4. Use cameras to teach people to take photographs. Make records of the work of each person. These have proved invaluable, particularly when we have made colour transparencies. These can be produced at a later date as an actual session—the puppets of course will look marvellous on celluloid—and provide a stimulating study. Slides may be taken of scenes from the show, and then the whole story can be retold. Be sure to photograph the puppeteers as well as the puppets.

Cine film can be taken as well, though of course this is very much more expensive. But one should be prepared to budget carefully and not to rely on traditional materials only, if the activities they offer are too limited to be effective.

5. Also try video equipment. This is easily accessible from TV rental firms if it is not already gathering dust in store cupboards. Used with groups of people who are mentally handicapped this could provide marvellous opportunities to help them find out more about what they look like and how they relate to others, in addition to its artistic potential. If there is one thing handicapped people have experience of it is television, so it makes obvious sense to use this familiarity creatively.

I have worked with groups of people with all kinds of equipment. Someone has been responsible for the plug and the switch at the wall, someone else for the switch on the machine, someone else did something else and the shared responsibility fostered confidence as well as involvement.

Music

The therapy that lies in music can have a far-reaching effect upon the development of children who bear the handicaps of mental impairment, emotional disturbance or physical disability. Over wide ranges of childhood pathology, age, social and economic background, under almost all conditions of special education, institutional or clinical care, this broad assertion holds true.

Music is a universal experience in the sense that all can share in it; its fundamental elements of melody, harmony, and rhythm appeal to, and engage their related psychic functions in each one of us. Music is also universal in that its message, the content of its expression, can encompass all heights and depths of human experience, all shades of feeling. It can lead or accompany the psyche through all conditions of inner experience, whether these be superficial and relatively commonplace or profound and deeply personal.

That the cultural inheritance of music is endowed with countless gifts for every human being is common knowledge, but for those children with whom we are concerned in this book the "gifts" that music holds are so important that they demand our special consideration. Because these children are mentally or emotionally or physically handicapped — or as is very often the case, multiply handicapped—each one is isolated from the course and content of normal human life to a particular extent. Frequently the handicapped child is unable to assimilate life's experiences; he may be confused because he fails to interpret them, he may even misinterpret them. He may have little or no faith in the capacities of his own psyche. His responsiveness to life may be crippled by fear or anxiety; he may live in a vortex of emotion or, conversely, his consciousness can be so remote that it is concerned only with distorted fragments of the realities of existence. Severe physical disability may have confined him from birth, narrowing his developmental contact with life, his communicative difficulties denying him all expectation of competence and fulfilment, his dependency demoralizing him. For children such as these music may have become a world of cogent, activating experience.

For the child who is intellectually impaired, music and musical activities can be vivid, intelligible experiences that require no abstract thought. For the emotionally immature or disturbed child the experience of the emotional language of music is inviting; the self-subsistence of its melodies and forms provides security for him. Musical activity can motivate the physically disabled child to use his limbs or voice expressively; its rhythmic-melodic structures then support his activity and induce an order in his control that promotes coordination. Music therefore becomes a sphere of experience, a means of intercommunication and a basis for activity in which handicapped children can find freedom in varying degrees, from the malfunctions that restrict their lives. As such, music possesses inherent capacitites for effecting a uniquely significant contact with handicapped children and for providing an experiential ground for their engagement, their personality development, their integration—both individually and socially. To the extent to which music achieves this it become music therapy; in practice, the range of expression of music as art, and the structural constitution of music as an artistic discipline are directly involved. (*Therapy in Music for Handicapped Children* by Paul Nordoff and Clive Robbins)

This very warmly observant book, from whose introduction I have quoted so extensively, has proved very useful to me. Although the authors talk about "musically-supported activities" however, they do not mention puppets. What they do say is that music as a medium may at times be almost too fluid for children who are extremely handicapped, and have to be incorporated as music-melodrama.

We have already seen profoundly handicapped children using musical instruments as sound effects. These sound effects have been used to reinforce action and character, in other words to build up atmosphere. Further effects and an even more enriching experience could be created by working with a musician or music therapist.

Music has no universal symbolism, it can only be interpreted by the personal inner language of each listener. Yet however elusive music may appear, the aural memory of most people is very strong. A handicapped person may retain little information about ordinary everyday facts, and yet at the same time remember almost every word of the song at the top of the hit parade! We shall say more about this later on.

It is possible to buy a wonderful array of percussion instruments, most of them originating, like our shadow puppets, in the Far East: bamboo chimes, mother of pearl chimes, blocks for tapping, wooden ribs for scraping, metal and wood hollow shapes for beating. There are also numbers of bells and bars, simple whistles, drums and tambourines. Make a collection of these instruments and have them in use alongside the puppets. Incorporate noise makers too in the costumes of the puppets—bells, rattling beads, jangling pieces of metal, shells etc.

Single records are usually just the right length for a puppet show. There you have a ready-made musical structure to limit the distance you can wander as a performer in the early stages. Nursery rhymes, children's songs and pop songs can all provide the basis for a first show, and all have the advantage that you will be starting off in a familiar medium.

Although my own musical experience has been limited more or less to the use of these simple songs, it has led me to make more investigations into the way we speak and the kinds of speech rhythms we use. Once the rhythm of a foreign language is mastered it becomes easier to speak and to memorise. The rhythm of speech gives it an overall shape: when we see a square drawn on a piece of paper we are seeing a complete figure, not four lines, and in the same way when hearing a melody we perceive the *whole* thing and not just a series of unconnected sounds. If we break speech down into very basic rhythmic structures it becomes possible for quite extensive speeches to be understood by the handicapped puppeteers or audience. See illustration on page 152.

It is true that this stressed basic rhythm is not something we

often hear in real-life speech, but art can take an aspect of
reality to highlight it in a special way. Poetry is only words, like
prose, but the words are used in a special way to say certain
things without the constraints of everyday prose. In
encouraging people to express themselves through artistic
media, one may indeed have to forego correctness in favour of
freedom of expression. I have often made up simple scripts
from the actual phrases used by mentally handicapped
children. By making them into songs, chants and rhythmic
prose we have made the use of words an exciting experience.

If you are working with people who are able actually to
learn lines it is important that everyone learns *all* the lines first
and you sort out who is going to say what later. Learning of
lines can take place with the whole group sitting down clapping
out the rhythm, and coming in with the words on the right
beat—in the way a dancer has to count himself in. This may be
done with or without puppets at first but, of course, the aim is
to enable the person to speak through the puppet.

Puppets in speech therapy
Therapists are often keen to use puppets in language
programmes *apart* from the art experience. It is, however,
important to remember that there is a difference between using
puppets as visual aids and using them as an expressive art-
form. Puppets can be both the means and motivation for
communication, they can be successfully used according to the
tastes of the people concerned. But whatever the case, the aim
should be that the whole person, the whole creative person,
should be able to use the medium. One occupational therapist
said to me recently ''Language is *everything*'' and of course it is,
verbal and non-verbal, and one should beware of looking at a
language problem in terms of speech only.

So if you are a speech therapist for instance, interested in
using puppets in your clinical sessions, try to encourage the
patient to use puppets fully, in the ways we have been
examining throughout the book. If you are using puppets only
as visual aids towards some other end, you run the risk of
falling between two stools: the puppet experience will be
fruitless and the language goals unattained. If on the other

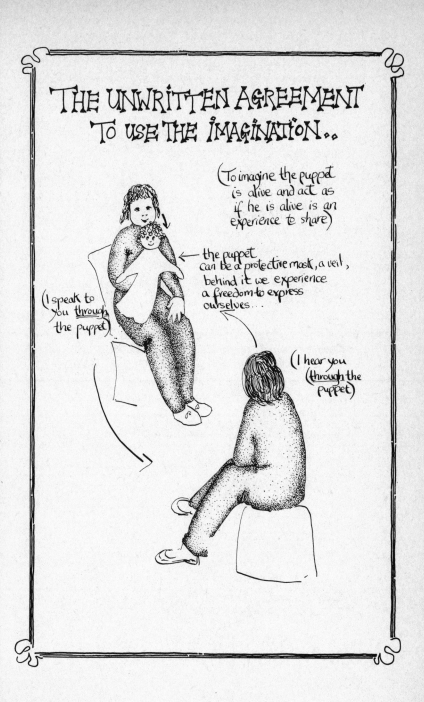

Breaking speech down to rhythmic structure.

```
          1  2   1   2   3  4  1, 2, 3,
F.N.   Hallo Mister Lazy, How are you ?
          1    2      1 2 3    4
M.2.   I'm alright Feathery Nose
          1    2   3    4    1   2   3    4
F.N.   What a mess you look a mess you
          1  2    1    2    3
       never brush' your' hair.
```

Simple tunes. Every attempt should be made to record tunes - however simple and however repetitive.

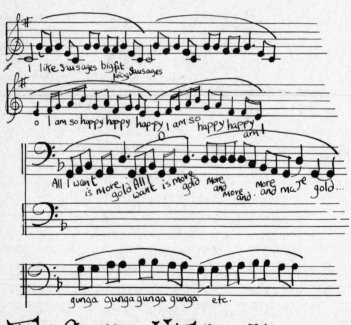

I like sausages big fat juicy sausages

o I am so happy happy happy I am so happy happy I am

All I want is more gold All I want is more gold More and more and more and more gold...

gunga gunga gunga gunga   etc.

THE SPEECH NOTEBOOK...

hand you look towards the experience of the *whole* person—the freedom of the individual to express himself better in a complete way, which may or may not be evident immediately in terms of speech results—eventually artistic freedom will affect him in every aspect of his being.

Some exercises
Object recognition

1. Use a Tubby-type puppet with wired hands to hold objects. The therapist controls the puppet. Have a number of objects of normal sizes: toothbrushes, hairbrush, cup, spoon etc. Fix them into the hand of the puppet, and ask the patient to "help" the puppet to use the object. The moment she shows the correct response make the puppet move. Gradually the proportion of physical activity by the patient will increase but at first be prepared to do most of the work yourself, through the puppet.

2. Have a set of *identical objects* to the group above. Place one in the hand of the puppet and demonstrate to the child that you want her to find the equivalent one in his collection. The objective should be for the child to match object to object.

3. Introduce objects of the same function but of different sizes or colours, and play the same game, this time matching object to function.

Large doll play

Since a large puppet is being used in the above exercise, we are already involved in large doll play. But the puppet has advantages over the ordinary doll. A glove puppet can pick up objects, pour, lift, act out drinking, use simple toys all by means of the hand concealed inside the body, whereas the doll can do these things only with visible interference. With the puppet, you may be able to encourage the patient to learn to play independently if she is sufficiently interested. If a person can understand the significance of objects or actions only if the therapist or another adult is actually working at the same activity then the puppet, as an "extra" character, can help to underline the value of the activity and to direct the attention of the child.

1. Repeat all the above activities, but encourage more and more interaction with the puppet. Teach the child to use the hands of the puppets by coming around behind the puppet with you.

2. Play a copying game. You drink. Puppet drinks. Child drinks etc.

3. Extend the use of common objects to more unusual objects—an umbrella for example. Keep a number of similar but not necessarily identical objects in the room to be searched out by you, the child and the puppet . . . for making special collections.

4. Make collections of objects for use by the child or puppet. Select them in categories: colours, objects, things for eating, dressing, playing, carpentry, cooking, cars, animals, birds, large things, small things.

6. Give the large puppet a shopping bag. Help her to collect the particular category of things she is interested in; or ask for a different thing each time but have the categories of article kept in their own places so that the child may fetch what is required—eg. "Get me something red; fetch me a car; fetch the puppet a drinking cup."

6. Make a giant mouth puppet and ask the child to put the things she collects into the mouth . . . the puppet eats rubbish. See how to make this special puppet.

This puppet is designed to reward activity in two different ways: the first reward comes from the sound of the object hitting the hollow tin base of the puppet, the second from the therapist allowing a sweet to drop down one or other of the hand tubes, into the hand of the child (page 155).

7. Use the Tubby puppet again. He has three buckets in front of him, all different colours. Give the child one object of a similar pair. Tubby covers the other object with one of the buckets and then moves all three about . . . Have a sweet slipped beneath the bucket concealing the object. Stop

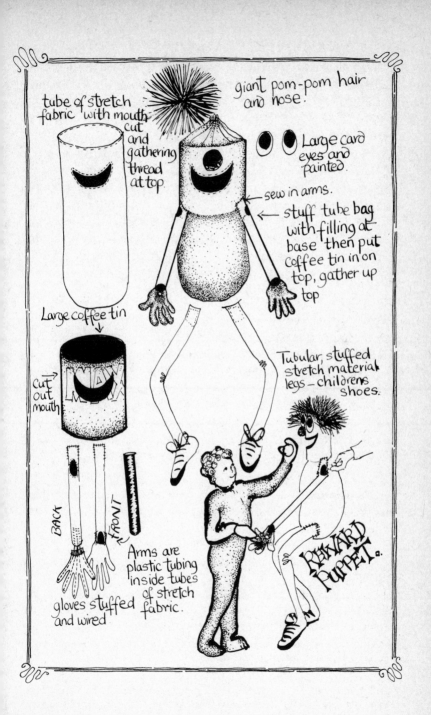

tube of stretch fabric with mouth cut and gathering thread at top.

giant pom-pom hair and nose.

Large card eyes and painted.

sew in arms.

stuff tube bag with filling at base then put coffee tin in on top, gather up top

Large coffee tin

cut out mouth

Tubular, stuffed stretch material legs – childrens shoes.

BACK

FRONT

Arms are plastic tubing inside tubes of stretch fabric.

gloves stuffed and wired

REWARD PUPPET.

the movement, the child has to find the object. If this
becomes too easy, play the game with buckets of the same
colour.

Small doll play

Build the scenario out of small cardboard boxes. Make it as
colourful and as varied in texture as you can. Have treasure
hunts, chases, act out nursery rhymes—*Three Blind Mice*, for
example. Place the whole scene in front of a large mirror.

Avoid speaking at first, simply act with the child using little
finger puppets, and show what is required. Later on add
concise verbal instruction.

Body image

This game should ideally be played with the Charig Puppets
SIMON. The puppet comes apart, so lay all his features out on
the floor: hands, feet, eyes, mouth, nose, ears, arms, legs etc.
Be sure they are all clearly visible.

Ask the children to find their own physical features one at a
time and then to put the puppet together piece by piece.
Then you will be able to play "Simon says" or sing a song
like, "Head, shoulder, knees and toes."

If you do not have a Charig Puppets SIMON, you can make a
simple version instead—but of course it is not as useful (page
158).

Draw around a head and body on paper. Strengthen with a
wooden baton. Cut out thick paper features. Use paper
fasteners to attach the features to the body and head. Facial
details can be fixed temporarily with Blu-tak.

Position concepts

Maurice Mouse is a useful little puppet to use to teach
positional concepts. Use him for crawling on the table or
underneath the furniture. You might combine this with role
playing the cat as well—and performing *Pussycat, Pussycat where
have you been?*, with a child taking one of the parts. A chase is
always popular.

When role-playing has become of interest, it will be time to
introduce a simple booth (eg. the table) and a selection of

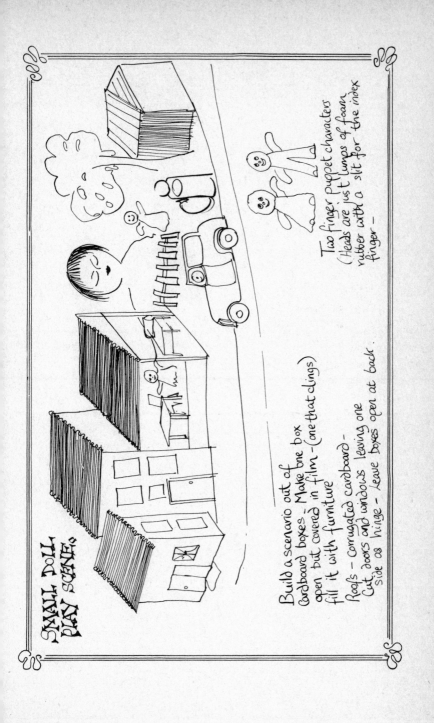

SMALL DOLL PLAY SCENE.

Build a scenario out of cardboard boxes. Make one box open but covered in Film - (one that clings) fill it with furniture

Roofs - corrugated cardboard -

Cut doors and windows leaving one side as hinge - leave boxes open at back.

Two finger puppet characters (Heads are just lumps of foam rubber with a slit for the index finger -

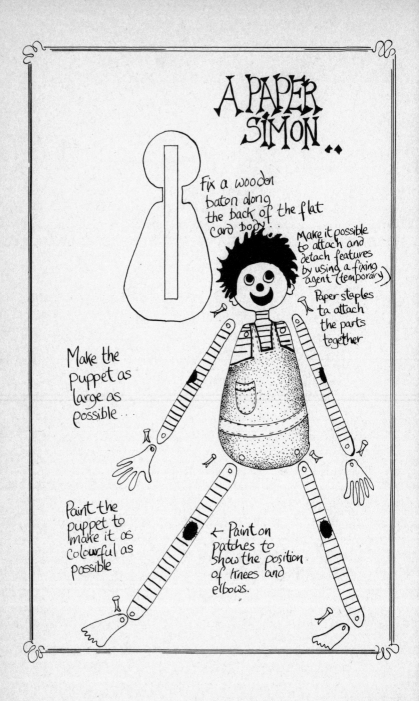

A PAPER SIMON..

Fix a wooden baton along the back of the flat card body.

Make it possible to attach and detach features by using a fixing agent (temporary)

Paper staples ta attach the parts together

Make the puppet as large as possible...

Paint the puppet to make it as colourful as possible

← Paint on patches to show the position of knees and elbows.

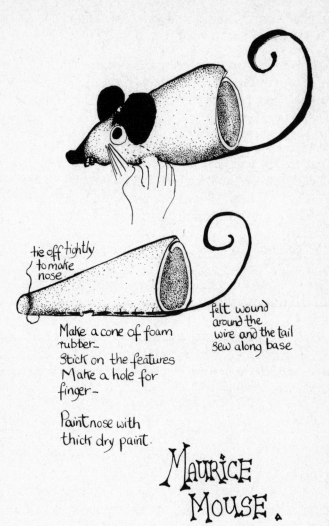

tie off tightly
to make
nose.

felt wound
around the
wire and the tail
sew along base

Make a cone of foam
rubber.
Stick on the features
Make a hole for
finger.

Paint nose with
thick dry paint.

MAURICE
MOUSE.

puppets to act out special scenes. It might also be time for the child to see a puppet show.

Another look at the previous notes on animation will offer special opportunities to work in two dimensions.

Further work with puppets may be suggested by the following letter from a teacher in a special unit for mentally handicapped children. The teacher had recently added the Charig puppet SIMON to her class.

> Simon is a *huge* success. We call him Simon Cork and he sits supported by his elastic on a special chair. At present he has a table before him with all the necessary cutlery and plates etc. He gets so cross if the knife and fork are the 'wrong' way round! To extend vocabulary he now wears:
> *Ear*-ring;
> A silver chain *neck* lace;
> Badges (on his *chest*) bracelet;
> Watch on his *wrist*; bandage (on his *ankle*!);
> Pair of child's spectacles which just balance nicely on his *nose*!
>
> His hair is sometimes arranged as a beard!
>
> I lent him to one of the infant classes (five- to six-year-olds) and they measured him and produced a great deal of interesting written work.
>
> I have found Simon extremely useful for art work and our paintings have taken on quite a different look! The children look at him carefully and then try to reproduce him with paint and crayon. One child got his ears and matched them to make sure they were the same size.
>
> We've discovered that our big toes go together, and our thumbs! Our elbows and knees bend like Simon's, and of course we can look sad or miserable!
>
> I've been really delighted with the class's response and naturally it has also given me much pleasure. Thank you very much!

After a performance at a school for severely handicapped children, one of the teachers hurried her class away because they all wanted to paint pictures of what they had seen. Later on a search party was sent out to find me before I left in my car, because they had a surprise for me. To my amazement, laid out on the floor were twenty paintings, some of them detailed, some of them exhilarated splashes of colour, of which the artists would explain the meaning—the figurative meaning—putting me right if I interpreted wrongly. The teacher was delighted by the response of her class—some children who were normally reticent or who had little language, were not only emotionally stimulated by the morning but were able to express themselves intellectually afterwards: their art had content but they also attempted to verbalise what they had seen. This reminded me of something else I believe: that the truly creative act sparks off another creative act—one acts as the impulse for the next.

Special problems
Although there have been many instances already in this book where the profoundly mentally handicapped have been involved with puppets, it might be an idea to describe more fully the situation of many of these people.

Although there are clubs for the more able mentally handicapped, the social life of the profoundly disabled is very limited indeed. There are those who question whether such people really need to have a ''social life'' at all. So how can the teaching of art help the profoundly handicapped person in need of special care?

If one is convinced of the potential of every person however handicapped, his creativity and his ability to communicate and form human relationships, what guidelines are necessary in order to offer creative experience?

1. Depending on the stage of development of the person, it is probable that he will appear to enjoy much physical play and water play with the puppets, where rewards are sensual more than intellectual. *However, it is still important to offer entertainment in the way of music, and simple dramatic performances using masks, props or puppets.*
2. Integrate profoundly handicapped people in the audience with able helpers. Place seating/wheelchairs according to hearing or seeing capabilities.

3. Prepare your audience individually, as far as possible, for what you are going to do.

A visit I made to a holiday resort for people requiring special care illustrates what I mean. There were about ten guests and the same number of staff. I arrived, set up my equipment in the gymnasium and performed. But the whole thing seemed to fall very flat. After the show, the organiser and I went over what had happened, and we agreed that the following week I should arrive much earlier and have lunch with the guests and helpers and get to know some of them first. This I did, and after the meal, showed everyone individually the puppets (there was an age range of about six to forty years). The staff, most of whom were voluntary, encouraged the children to handle or look at the puppets. When everyone was assembled for the performance (this time we set up in the staff-room, which was cosier and had a much lower ceiling) I suggested to the helpers that they reinforce all the puppets did by shouting, singing or pointing, helping the guests to clap or point as well—in fact, taking each person through the experience physically. I reassured the audience that I would not lose concentration and that they could be as active as they liked, as long as all they did was concentrated on the action.

One might have expected the guests to have been thoroughly distracted by what was going on around them, but in fact most of them were reported afterwards to have sat very still watching the booth intently. One or two smiled at some of the happenings, and one lady kept saying, ''Dollies'' over and over again.

4. Those children whose behaviour is erratic or destructive (intentionally or unintentionally)—they are sometimes called hyperactive—are best left wandering during the show but watched.

There was one child who swung from the wall bars while I was performing, and then came right up to the front of the shadow booth to touch the shadows. I held her in front of me with both arms wrapped around in a very firm embrace—she was show-ing a genuine interest in the puppets, but seemed unable to express her excitement in the conventional somewhat more confined way. Later during the glove puppets show, she occupied herself with throwing scraps of waste paper through the stage-opening, and became a distraction.

A greater freedom of movement than usual should be permissible in the audience, as conventions are meaningless to the most handicapped. More active people should be allowed to move around, but should be watched and possibly followed. I always ask for a helper to be back stage with me to keep an eye on the equipment.

I have actually run around pursuing a child who is hyperactive, just to keep him still long enough to watch the puppet on my hand. When I finally caught up with him, the puppet sang a song to the little boy which he continued to sing for the rest of the day.

Sadly, once a head of a school put all the ''noisy'' children beside the door so that they could be taken away if they interrupted too much. Loud strange noises and unusual movements or antics are something a performer for the handicapped has to endure, but it becomes less a problem of endurance and simply part of the character of an audience—a very positive personality with whom to be friends: the puppeteer with the audience.

5. If anyone in the audience uses sign language, it is important to have someone interpreting and paraphrasing.

In one hospital school I visited the children had learnt Makaton. For the day on puppetry, the children were divided into groups of about seven or eight, each child with a helper who knew some basic signs. The first part of the project involved the children in using the SIMON puppet, and then in learning the characters they were to see later in performance.

I showed the children the incomplete body of SIMON and they took turns pulling out parts of his body from the shopping bag, identifying them if they could, and attaching them in the right places. Applause followed, and also ''good boy'' or ''good girl'' in Makaton. The SIMON game made a lively start to each group—some children who were more lively tried to put the whole puppet together on their own.

After this I told the story of the main puppet show. I showed them the puppets at the same time, and also gave them the signs for the type of character—"good man", "bad man" etc. By concentrating on the characters first, the children quickly grasped the dramatic interaction and were also able to join in with their part of action: recognising and participating with the particular characters. The performance of the show was to be a week after the workshops sessions, and the preparation paid off. Many of the children remembered the puppets and the characters they played.

Although the children were quite bright and receptive, it was however the end of the summer play scheme and most of the helpers had been at a party the night before and were somewhat the worse for wear. They were unable to give the support their charges needed to help them watch the actual performance. The show, without much collective audience response, went by quickly.

Disappointed, I decided to let the children play with the puppets themselves, so I asked for chairs to be taken into the booth and let the children take turns in climbing in and holding different puppets up for the audience. They needed no encouragement! I peeped in at the side and saw to my surprise a boy holding up the "bad man" to the playboard, and with the other hand, his whole expression "acting", signing "bad man, bad man, bad man!" It was the only time I had ever seen spontaneous signing in a mentally handicapped child.

Multiply handicapped people

Many mentally handicapped people have an additional physical handicap, so although this book is not about people who are physically handicapped it may be useful to look at some of the problems in making puppets available to people with additional problems.

First, special attention may have to be given to adjusting hand grips and controls. In some cases whole puppets may have to be designed with a particular person in mind. If a person is mobile but unable to stand for any length of time, it may be necessary to design puppets especially for the wheelchair. Wheelchairs—electric or manual—provide

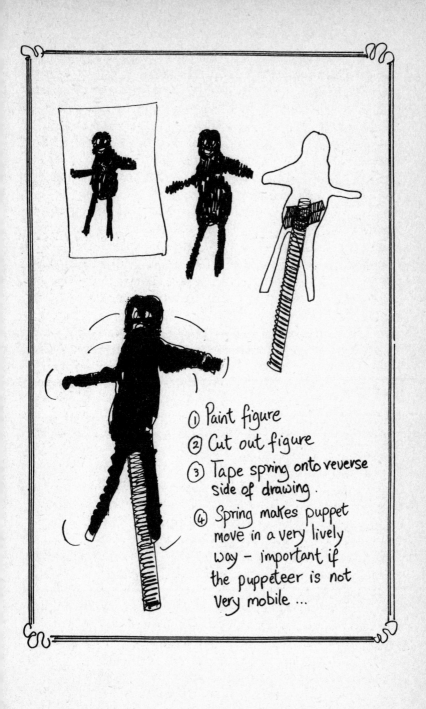

1. Paint figure
2. Cut out figure
3. Tape spring onto reverse side of drawing.
4. Spring makes puppet move in a very lively way – important if the puppeteer is not very mobile ...

marvellous scope for gadgetry. Recently some students designed special puppets for people more or less confined to wheelchairs and there seemed to be no end to the possi- bilities—they came up with ideas ranging from tremendously elaborate Heath Robinson affairs with weights and pulleys, to simple rod puppets. It was agreed that for the mentally alert but chronically physically disabled a challenge would be attractive, so the puppets were designed to do amusing but simple things—drinking out of a bottle, or hitting someone—with the mechanics made as interesting as possible.

One boy who came to some of my sessions was about fourteen years old, severely subnormal, with little spoken language, and almost completely incapacitated by muscular dystrophy: he had only a little movement in his neck and fingers and mouth. With help, he made a number of puppets, and especially enjoyed a paper-puppet man on a spring which was made directly from his own painting of a man—"me" he said. The most successful puppets, however, were a selection made for him to use on the overhead projector. He initiated the activity by telling me what characters he wanted: he made attempts to say the words—"Pleece, pleece!" "Gooh mah", "Bah mah". His train of thought usually ran in the direction of ghosts or the latest cops and robbers television programme.

I made a selection of simple paper puppets, which the boy worked with drinking straws. The projector was placed on a low table, exactly in line with his hands when they were resting on his lap. He was able to shift his weight to get himself into the best position for using his fingers, and at times he would allow his body to drop far enough to allow him to use his teeth to grip with.

He enjoyed making the big images on the wall, and this instant reward for effort was obviously important, for his concentration increased from just a few minutes watching, to telling a long involved story about a man and his car. The car was stolen, the police went after the thief—then there was a fire and the fire engine had to come. He had quite a good memory and remembered the details of the story so he kept on repeating them, adding extra details and changing bits around to suit himself.

The very first time I asked this boy to tell a story, he took a deep breath and then started to make a series of sounds in exactly the intonation one would use to repeat a tale to a child. *"Once* upon a *time* . . . and they *all* lived *happily ever after"* . . . He did not use words at all—just the "tune" of the tale. (When he tried to use words, real ones, the tune disappeared as he struggled.) He was an imaginative child, who had always enjoyed watching performances, and now he was prepared to use puppets to perform to me. He enjoyed singing and he would throw back his head and wordless sounds came out of his mouth. In order to "tell' the story he moved the puppets around on the flat screen, became excited, moved them around until they fell off at the side and then found another character or prop to continue. The puppets in short gave him an alternative language, they caught the fluidity of his emotions and the puppets became *words*. The lengths of the sessions continued to increase—some lasting over an hour—and the stories themselves became more concentrated and artistically exciting.

Social Training

Social training is an unfortunate term—to refer to someone as "trainable" hints at circus antics or a dog show. Somewhere in the most unresponsive being is a person who is not a "patient", who should not even have come to be a "problem", but is part of society. From the moment a person is conceived—even unborn—he is a member of society with certain rights—moral and legal. As a young child he has a right to expect his environment to adapt to his needs and only as his own dependency lessens is he expected to begin to adapt to society: his awareness of the adaptations necessary develops from early care he receives. Where early loving care is not available his capacities are lost and talents are left undeveloped. Instead of trust, defensiveness develops—even in the very young.

Thus many young people slightly handicapped have a very low opinion of themselves, and this poor self-image contributes to behaviour problems, leading to relationship problems.

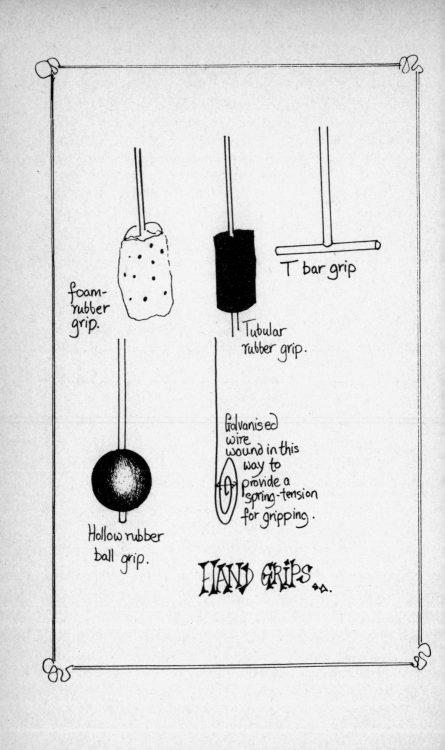

foam-
rubber
grip.

T bar grip

Tubular
rubber grip.

Galvanised
wire
wound in this
way to
provide a
spring-tension
for gripping.

Hollow rubber
ball grip.

HAND GRIPS.

Social training—teaching a person to be adaptive—is not enough without an emotional, empathetic relationship to provide the framework for the training. The ability to adapt can only develop out of an environment which holds respect for individuality and cherishes idiosyncrasy in those we care about so that it may be converted into creative expression. The confidence which comes from knowing one can be a pleasure to others, that one is accepted and loved, gives stability to a person and enables him to adapt to the different circumstances he is likely to meet.

Social training should involve every aspect of a person's life and his part in the community: relationships, marriage, sexuality. Social training should start as soon as possible affirming the young person as a first-class and not a second-class citizen. Social training through art should be an opportunity to examine values and not only to receive values as they are handed out.

Following are a number of basic scripts for puppet plays that may be used in this critical approach to social training. They deal with the following themes:

Relationships
> The responsibility of having a job and being paid for it; The vulnerability of mentally handicapped people. From whom can they expect help and support?
> Handling relationships with the opposite sex—public behaviour and social norms; some public street signs;
> Men have to be domesticated too;
> Sex and contraception.

The puppets should be simple glove puppets and the plays can be performed either at a table, with a small group of people, or with the puppeteers concealed, with a larger group of people. The puppets have to be involved with the slides projected on to a screen and the overhead projector. I suggest that the episodes be treated separately on different occasions, allowing plenty of time for questions and repetition of key moments.

Props should be made with care, so that they do not fall

down at the wrong moment—stick Velcro on to the bases. Taping a weight—a small block of wood—into the bottom of each box will make them more manageable by the puppet.

At work
Freddie comes on to playboard and piles up some boxes. He is in a hurry, and as he rushes off they all fall down again. He turns round, sees they have fallen.

FREDDIE   Silly stupid boxes, I'm in a hurry!

He piles them up again, they all fall down. He kicks them out the way and runs out.

                      Stupid boxes!

Enter Boss—friendly with glasses and smile. Sees the boxes.

BOSS   Who left these like this? What a mess! Who was it—was it that Freddie? Where has he gone? Freddie! Freddie!

FREDDIE   (*Entering*) What's that? What is it? Who's calling? I want to be off. I'm meeting my girl-friend Sally. Oh it's you, Boss!

BOSS   Yes it is.

FREDDIE   Well, I'm here for my money.

BOSS   Your what?

FREDDIE   My money!

BOSS   You want your money? What for?

FREDDIE   For tidying.

BOSS   Tidying what?

FREDDIE   I've been tidying the boxes like you told me to do.

BOSS   Look at the boxes, they're all a mess . . . What do you think, everyone—has he done his job properly, are the boxes tidy? Who left them in a mess, everyone? You have work to do, Freddie?

FREDDIE   Yes, Boss.

BOSS   Right then, do it and do it properly, right?

FREDDIE   Right.

Exit Boss.

FREDDIE   He's gone. I'd better get on and do it
             properly.

He piles them up again in a hurry, they all fall down on his head with a crash.

             Owww! I'd better take it easy.

Sings (to tune of Mulberry Bush)

             This is the way I pile up the boxes etc.
             On a Friday afternoon.
             I must learn to do my job properly etc.
             By a Friday afternoon.
             That's better, now I really have finished.

BOSS   Fine—now here's your money, Freddie.
             Don't spend it all at once.

FREDDIE   I'm taking my girl-friend Sally out.

Freddie meets someone who doesn't like him

FREDDIE   I've got my money. There, I'll put it into
             my pocket—it'll be safe there. I'm going
             to take my Sally out tonight.

In sneaks the Punk and pinches the pay-packet out of Freddie's pocket.
Freddie finds the money is missing and then rushes off to find a stick.

             Help, help I've been robbed—wait I'll get
             a stick—I'll bray 'im . . . I'll beat his
             head in—I'll knock his block off . . .

Comes back in with the stick, meanwhile the Policeman has come in.
Freddie crashes into him.

POLICEMAN   Hey—what's going on!

FREDDIE   You stole my money!

POLICEMAN   No I didn't.

FREDDIE   You did, you did!

POLICEMAN   Now then, just you calm down.

FREDDIE   You took my money—he did, didn't he,
             everyone? He didn't? Oh it's the
             Policeman!

POLICEMAN   Yes, that's right. Why don't you tell me
             what has been going on. And put that
             stick down. *You* don't go knocking
             people's heads off. I'll catch the man who
             stole your money.

Exit Freddie with Policeman. Punk comes up—stands around—Policeman creeps up on Punk—Punk creeps away. Policeman tries again and again and eventually succeeds.

POLICEMAN   There's your money Freddie—now no more sticks. It's *my* job to catch criminals.

FREDDIE   Thank you, Policeman.

A night out with Sally

Sally is dancing—Freddie goes up and tries to kiss her. She pushes him away.

SALLY   Not with all these people watching.

FREDDIE   You don't mind, do you, everyone?

SALLY   I mind—kissing's for private.

FREDDIE   Come on—let's go outside then.

SALLY   Let's dance.

FREDDIE   All right—afterwards then—then I'll kiss you.

SALLY   I don't mind afterwards in private. I like dancing.

FREDDIE   I only like dancing with you.

They stop and have a drink together

SALLY   I like doing everything with you, Freddie.

FREDDIE   You don't like kissing, do you? Want to go for a walk?

SALLY   It's too dark to go out walking.

FREDDIE   I'll take care of you.

They kiss each other

FREDDIE   I want to go to the toilet.

SALLY   You'll have to cross your legs then—you can't go here.

FREDDIE   I'm crossing my legs, I still want to go to the toilet. I'm off there behind that tree.

Sally runs away, Posh Lady comes out from behind tree screaming and beating Freddie with her umbrella

LADY   Nasty dirty man! (*Exit*)

SALLY   (*Laughing*) Serves you right—told you to wait and go to the proper toilet!

FREDDIE   I haven't been yet—there's the toilets there.

Two doors are in sight—one with female figure on the door, other with a

male. He rushes into the one marked female because it is nearer—out pops
Lady again screaming.

FREDDIE	Whoops, wrong one!
SALLY	You should have gone into that one.

Freddie comes back after going into the right one

SALLY	It's all right in the dark.
FREDDIE	I'm taking care of you.
SALLY	You can kiss me or do anything here now. No one's watching now, are they?
FREDDIE	Anything? I'm not doing anything? I'll kiss you but that's all, see?
SALLY	I can go and dance with someone else—they'll kiss me and *everything*.
FREDDIE	That's not fair—because it's me that wants to marry you.
SALLY	You haven't asked me yet—and I haven't said yes—and if you'll only kiss me—Well?
FREDDIE	I'm going off home, I'm off working in the morning.
SALLY	Just a kiss then . . .

At the Centre

FREDDIE	Will you marry me, Sally?
SALLY	I don't know.
FREDDIE	Tell her to marry me everyone!
SALLY	I'll tell you myself—NO.
FREDDIE	I'll give you a kiss.
SALLY	I'm busy learning to cook—I can make cakes. Mrs Brown is teaching me to make cakes—(*she throws some flour at Freddie*).
FREDDIE	(*Coughs*) Where's Sally? She's gone!
MRS BROWN	What on earth is happening here? Freddie!
FREDDIE	Sorry, Mrs Brown
MRS BROWN	You'll be sorry by the time you've cleared up all that flour—come on, you can get the brush.
FREDDIE	I'm going to marry Sally.

MRS BROWN	Does Sally know that?
FREDDIE	She knows—but she doesn't want to.
MRS BROWN	Now you've done that—you can fill that basin with water and do the washing-up.
FREDDIE	Me?
MRS BROWN	Yes—men who are going to be husbands have to learn all about that as well—

Freddie goes off.

SALLY	I'm learning to make cakes, Mrs Brown, because I'm going to be Mrs Freddie soon . . .
MRS BROWN	I don't think you'll be Mrs Anyone unless you learn to cook other things—leave that bowl of mixture to stand and have a look at the recipe cards.

They both go off.

FREDDIE	I've finished the washing-up—OOh what a great big bowl of mixture.

Sally creeps in behind him and makes him jump.

SALLY	Boo

Freddie falls into the cake mixture

FREDDIE	Help glug glug I've fallen in!
SALLY	You've spoilt my mixture—you've spoilt my cakes!
FREDDIE	I don't want you as my Mrs Freddie now!
SALLY	Oh Freddie—I'm sorry! I'm sorry! I'll kiss you better!
FREDDIE	Oh. We'll see then.
SALLY	I'll put the cakes in.
FREDDIE	Are they in now?
SALLY	Yes.
FREDDIE	How long do you have to wait for them to be ready?
SALLY	A few minutes on the clock.

The clock is facing the audience—the hands move round as Freddie and Sally have a cuddle.

SALLY	What's that smell—it's burning? You've spoilt my cakes again! It's your fault!

FREDDIE	If we were married we could kiss all the time. (*they laugh*)
SALLY	Yes!

They hug.

Visiting the Doctor

DOCTOR	So you are going to be married?
BOTH	Yes.
SALLY	Mrs Brown told me to come and find out about babies.
DOCTOR	Well, you know how babies are made?
FREDDIE	I know.
SALLY	But how do you *unmake* babies?
DOCTOR	Unmake babies?
FREDDIE	Stop them popping out.
DOCTOR	Sally, what happens to someone if they are having a baby?
SALLY	You get fat.
DOCTOR	And do you know why that is?
SALLY	The baby's growing bigger inside.
DOCTOR	Here are some photographs of that baby.

Slides of the unborn child are shown on the screen.

SALLY	OOh
FREDDIE	It is dark in there where the baby is, isn't it?
DOCTOR	It is dark—and the baby is growing in secret—but it's nice to have photographs to see how he's getting on.
SALLY	He looks like a real baby.
DOCTOR	He *is* a real baby—a real little person in the dark, and a bit of a secret—but he is real. Now, Sally, you want to know how to *unmake* a baby—is that right?
SALLY	Yes.
DOCTOR	How do you think that can be done, Freddie?
FREDDIE	Don't know.
DOCTOR	Why do you want to stop a little chap like that popping out—as you said.

SALLY	Nappies, and feeding—and in case the baby is sick and . . .
FREDDIE	Babies aren't like dolls—they *want* things.
DOCTOR	They take a lot of caring for. And you will be trying to take care of each other—
SALLY	I'll be Mrs Freddie.
DOCTOR	Well—there are ways of "unmaking" babies—
FREDDIE	Good—
SALLY	My friend said there were too.
DOCTOR	You can scrape them out of the inside of you—and then the baby comes out in bits. Or you can suck the baby out and that also breaks him all up. Or you can poison him with salt—and that dries him up and burns him—but he is all in one piece . . .
FREDDIE	Does it hurt the baby?
DOCTOR	Would it hurt you to have to be "unmade" like that?
SALLY	It's cruel, I think.
DOCTOR	There are pills—but you have to remember to take them—or possibly an injection.
SALLY	I don't like having injections—can't he have it instead?
DOCTOR	Yes—it does seem as if women have to have everything done to *them*. There are things for men to use.
FREDDIE	From the barber's?
DOCTOR	You know about them do you? It is a good thing for men to do what they can because men also have to do half the work to make babies—shall we watch the screen again?

How babies are made (Using the overhead projector)

SALLY	When we go to bed . . .
DOCTOR	Babies have to be started off by something called sexual intercourse—this does not have to happen in bed—it could be anywhere—Freddie—you have a penis—

	Look at the picture.
FREDDIE	My willy.
DOCTOR	To have sexual intercourse your penis—goes hard and then you can push it into Sally—there in the picture.
SALLY	We've done that already, haven't we Freddie—a long time ago—
FREDDIE	We thought it would be all right because we weren't in bed and babies only come out in bed.
SALLY	It was nice.
DOCTOR	Now I have described your half of the work to make a baby, Freddie—what about Sally? Babies don't always happen after sexual intercourse. Look at the picture again—now then, inside Sally she produces an egg—one every month—
SALLY	Oooh—a baby?
DOCTOR	Not yet—watch the picture—the egg is produced and sometimes it is at the same time as having sexual inter-course—Freddie remember has his penis in there—look at the picture and out of there come the sperm—and they have in them what you need to make a baby too. So we have what in Sally?
SALLY	Egg.
DOCTOR	And what in you, Freddie?
FREDDIE	Sperm.
DOCTOR	Now to make a baby the two have to get together—and that is the beginning of it all—Look at the picture.
SALLY	It doesn't look like a baby.
DOCTOR	Do you know what this is? *(Holding a daffodil)*
SALLY	A daffodil.
DOCTOR	Do you know what this is? *(Holding a bulb)*
SALLY	It looks like an onion.
DOCTOR	Nearly. No—it's a daffodil bulb—it

doesn't look like a daffodil but if we plant it and then wait—without any doubt it will grow up into a lovely daffodil. Now this thing—the sperm from Freddie and the egg from you, Sally—make up something called an embryo—which is an early baby. It doesn't look like a baby—but given the chance it will grow into a lovely baby. BUT do you think you could take care of a baby after it is born?

SALLY   No.

FREDDIE   She's taking care of *me*.

DOCTOR   If we decide to unmake the baby—that hurts the baby—because we have to kill it. I have another idea. Remember that the baby cannot be made unless we have the sperm from Freddie and the egg from Sally. If either of those are missing—no baby.

DOCTOR   When Freddie uses the sheath—look at the picture—it stops the sperm from going to join with the egg. If Sally takes a certain kind of pill—that stops the egg from going to meet the sperm. If you want to change your mind one day to have a baby, to bring him up to be a grown-up like you, then you could use the sheath or the pill. But if you decide never to have children—*never*, then there is something else you can do. A little operation that you might have, Sally—to stop your eggs going to meet Freddie's sperm; or you, Freddie, to stop your sperm going to meet Sally's egg. Then there will be no babies—EVER.

SALLY   I'm afraid of operations—I don't like them.

DOCTOR   The decision to have an operation like this—is a very important one—you

	should go away and think about it together.
SALLY	But I don't like operations.
FREDDIE	I'll take care of you little Sally,
SALLY	You have the horrible operation.
FREDDIE	All right.
DOCTOR	That would be a very loving thing to do, Freddie. But off you go now and think about everything I have said and come back later and tell me what you would like me to do.

The last of these little puppet plays for social training is much the longest as the subject matter obviously demands longer treatment.

Simple puppet plays like this can clear up a great deal of confusion about complex subjects such as sex. There is often confusion about "sleeping together" "having sex" "having babies" "going to bed". But there is no reason why even the biological aspects of human sexuality, as well as the whole idea of marriage, may not be presented in a way that mentally handicapped people might understand, and role play with puppets before a small group of people can help them to learn.

In the play 'Visiting the doctor' two puppeteers are necessary.

Slides of the unborn baby can be back projected on to a small screen with the Puppet Doctor using the control. The screen should be large enough to include the whole group in the play, as onlookers but participating as much as possible.

The overhead projector can be used to demonstrate sexual intercourse (you may not think this necessary, but it is if you want to show the mechanics of ovulation, ejaculation, fertilization and the formation of the embryo). The back projection screen should also have slides to demonstrate the stages of development of the embryo into the recognisable unborn baby.

For all the plays, gradually build up scenes, allowing each person to take different roles. Initially, always include yourself as one of the actors, but the objective should be to have all the puppets and props worked by people who are mentally handicapped.

Change words freely into the speech idioms of each person, and keep repeating the plays as games, with puppets and props and visual aid equipment available.

Back-up material
Visit police stations, discos, factories, churches, hospitals, doctors. Make collections of photographs, maps, street signs and other objects.

When puppets are not popular

Recently I met a highly individual young mongol girl brought up by parents in their late middle-age with a penchant for the theatre. Their daughter had all the fussy qualities of a middle-aged spinster and at the same time a childish delight in what was amusing or moving in entertainment. Although mentally handicapped, her aesthetic sense had been developed by the care and teaching from her parents who were able to share their own interests with her.

A utilitarian view of art can do inestimable damage. Of course the ability to produce things for use is as important as producing things of beauty to be enjoyed—and where both these aspects of creativity are combined then one balances the other. Where one view over-balances the other, however, one of two things happens. Either art becomes art for its own sake, the so-called artist "doing his own thing" not gifted enough actually to communicate anything, art becomes alienated from the rest of society. *For most people it is necessary to be heard by others, and this is especially important in the mentally handicapped artist.* Or, on the other hand, the great test of the artist becomes whether he can produce something someone else can use; and then whether he can produce something *anyone* can use—thus personal intercommunication is ruled out. The opportunity for idiosyncrasies in design—personal design—is ruled out, and the best design becomes that produced by the most people to please the most people. The next step is to find that a machine can produce what is required, and people become operators or machinists.

Both these unbalanced views end up negating the person and

his potential to communicate, one by removing all structure and framework for self-expression, the other by building up too much structure and then simply slotting people into the mechanistic framework. Either way, art becomes meaningless, at best not really necessary for our lives, at worst a plain and simple waste of time and money.

Even a person who is mentally handicapped is affected by views such as these, so that puppetry, or any other art, seems irrelevant or babyish. Such narrow attitudes affect the individual's whole view of life. When someone rejects art because it is not useful, ask yourself some questions about that person. Is he unwilling to be involved in social activities, and ill at ease for any length of time with others? Is he unrelaxed and apparently unable to sit still for a length of time, listening or watching others? Is he best when put to work at repetitive tasks which are physically involving—sweeping, cleaning? Does he become agitated or uncomfortable when the routine is altered and for some reason he cannot get on with his usual work?

Philip, a mongol man of about thirty, used to be allowed to clean the school when some children who were profoundly handicapped came for their annual holiday. He would come in and sit down for his tea-break and explain what he was doing and how important it was that he did this work. He would listen politely to any other conversation, but any attempt to keep him after he had drunk his tea would upset him. He also became upset if someone wanted unexpectedly to use the room he was about to clean. On this occasion it was this puppeteer! Philip was told that the puppet-show was for everyone, and he was welcome to join in. But almost without registering this, he began again his solemn explanation of what he had to do and why it was so important to do it. When we insisted that he could have the time off with everyone else, Philip became more distressed at the thought of his time being wasted.

Inflexible and insensitive teaching had left Philip with a very confined attitude to life—handicapping him further. Art provides the opportunities to make personal choices and decisions, to think things through. This capacity enables us to be more flexible, more adaptive and therefore to have more control over our lives.

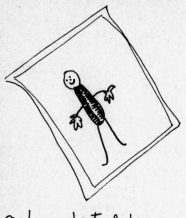

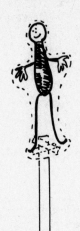

① Lay a sheet of clear acetate over white paper.

② Using special pens draw on the acetate

③ Cut figure out in the way indicated.

④ Cut a strip of acetate and cellotape onto figure...

A PUPPET FOR THE OVERHEAD PROJECTOR...

Exercises to encourage the capacity to adapt
Use the overhead projector,
the shadow screen,
a simple camera,
tape-recorder,
white paper,
clear acetate sheets,
pens for writing on film,
coloured acetate for changing colour of the light.

1. Ask each person in the group to draw a figure on a sheet of clear acetate placed on top of a piece of white paper (so that they can see what they are doing);
or, trace over ready-drawn figures (from a children's colouring book for example) helping each person to make his own choice of character.

2. Cut out the figures and tape them on to a strip of acetate to use as control.

So far everyone has passed from one medium to another, from drawing to animation.

3. Split each person one at a time from the main activity to: take a photograph, work the music on the tape-recorder, make a tape of the story, control the machinery. Ask who would like to work what?

4. Use the shadow screen—here work on a much larger scale. Give each person a piece of the coloured acetate to hold over the light bulb or to move across the screen. Ensure a repeated change of colour by taking one pair at a time, with the others watching. Make a light show.

5. Choose some suitable instrumental music—classical or rock. Imagine for example that you want to illustrate a fire. Put the music on at faster than the normal speed.

6. Imagine the scene using the different colours—the red glow, the embers, then change into blue and yellow and red for flames. Use dark chiffon-type material to swirl across the screen as smoke.

7. Behind the screen the group has to work as a team, but they must also become involved in the dramatic impact of the scene. Once again break up the activity with questions:

Who would like to work the red? Who would like to work the tape-recorder?

8. Introduce a man character. Allow each person to make a silhouette character on a horizontally placed rod—to allow the character to be pushed around and to turn somersaults. Take turns—each person acting the part of dancing in the fire according to the movement implied in the music. The introduction of the man puppet will encourage the group members to animate the flames. Try chasing with the flames, and knocking the man back.

9. Introduce very simple birds on rods—let them fly around trying to escape the flames.

Questions to ask

How will the fire die down?

Should it be put out?

What happens to fires?

Be ready to provide black silhouette fire-engines, hoses, blankets, water-buckets or rain clouds— depending where the discussion leads you!

The activity has been designed to encourage crossing over from one medium to another within the structured whole of the puppet show. Remember to include some of the group as audience at different times. It is simple enough to repeat exercises like this by altering the subject matter. You might include some aspects of social training in different puppet characters. It is important, though, to keep up the tension of the drama in order to carry along the less willing puppeteers.

Much unwillingness to work with puppets arises from a lack of confidence in a new situation. Among the intellectually more able, a fear of failure, self-consciousness, an awareness of their own clumsiness may well be involved. With such older and only mildly mentally handicapped children it is often effective to use larger puppets. Boys especially, and teenagers of both sexes, in my experience, enjoy the challenge of these. There is no need to be limited by scale, I have mixed up finger puppets with larger paper puppets and four- to seven-feet high rod puppets all in the same production. I have also mixed up actors with puppets nine feet high. The aim is to provide colourful, imaginative entertainment which would be attractive to the audience but also a challenge to perform.

The teenage years can be particularly difficult for teaching, and individual teenagers present particular problems. Young people at this age are both trying to express their individuality and at the same time submerging their identities into the crowd of their own peer group. Group identity provides the incentive for extravagantly exciting experiments — team games, competitive sports, fighting, vandalism, sexual experimentation. To counter the rejection of puppetry along with other conventional adult values, puppetry has to be presented appropriately.

The challenge in using large puppets also reinforces the ability of a person to be master of his puppet. To be physically in charge of what he is "giving life" to makes the experience more involving. A small child grows and as he develops he first of all gains control of his body before his imagination comes into play. Later on in teenagers who are backward imaginative growth must also be accompanied by simultaneous physical stimulation — which can be provided by the use of large puppets. These puppets have advantages over smaller ones when the capacity for fine motor control might be limited in clumsier children. The larger puppet is controlled by much larger movements — sweeps of the arms instead of light finger movements — giant strides on the floor instead of controlled arm movements.

Once I had an experience with a large aggressive boy who had a reputation for bullying. More by accident than judgement he ended up with the star part of a show — which was to be performed in a local village church at Easter time. The role he had to play was the Christ character — and he took that as a compliment, and made a beautiful puppet. The puppet was large and cumbersome and was supported by a pelvic belt—which was an advantage, as it meant that his legs were more or less tied together and his mobility reduced. For the Crucifixion scene I had intended simply to have the puppet with his arms outstretched, but the young puppeteer thought differently and for an entire morning he cut, stapled, tied and sliced away at cardboard and timber, and then to the envy of the rest of the class dragged through the door an enormously heavy Cross. During the play he tied the puppet to the Cross and then with great physical effort and tremendous endurance lifted it up and held it high in view of the congregation for the remaining twenty minutes of the performance. (His arms being fully occupied and his legs tied together rendered the lad harmless to the other boys and girls—but, of course, *that* was not the object of the exercise.)

These larger puppets obviously need more clothing than the small ones, and offer plenty of scope for large scale techniques.

1. *Fabric painting and dyeing:* stretch white cloth—sheeting, for example—over a frame. Paint on patterns with acrylic paint (not powder). Felt tips, paint sprays, or paint-on dyes can be used. Stick or sew on sequins, buttons or contrasting materials.

2. *Hands* may be made simply by drawing around the hands of each other, cutting the outline out of cardboard and attaching to the corners of the cloth.

3. *Colouring the face* can be done with paint. Hair can be made from wool—the latter can be washed and then set on rollers and dried into a rough style like human hair, though brushing out is more difficult and drying must be by heat from a drier.

Dressing and preparing the details of the puppet could provide a basis for an interesting session related to social training.

Subject matter for teenage plays should include plenty of fight scenes and love scenes. If a fight scene is not included, it will only be a matter of minutes before one breaks out. Having the scene to look forward to should pre-empt any otherwise disruptive activity.

Activity amongst teenagers is distinguished by certain characteristics: extremes of activity and lethargy, tension building leading to the release of tension after a period of concentration, and the release of tension giving rise to pleasure.

Many mentally handicapped young people are unable to sustain concentration for any length of time, so they miss the build-up of tension and the pleasure following—and the extremes of emotion involved in activity. The result is bland experience, marked by frustration, lack of achievement and boredom.

To capture a young person's imagination with an activity which is gripping, and a challenge which is realistic, could be the way to channel the potential for activity away from boredom to fulfilment.

Fear of puppets

Another reason for rejecting puppetry may be fear. Fear is usually expressed by averting the eyes away from the puppet, hiding the face or running away. It is usually the three-dimensional puppets which cause the most anxiety.

Ways of combating the anxiety:

Use shadow puppets initially. Never thrust a puppet into a person's face.

It would be useful to re-read the notes on *Hilary the Green Witch* (page 96). Remember that puppetry involves the willing agreement between puppeteers and audience to speak through the imagination by the use of the puppets. It is not one person trying to fool another. Even the most marvellous conjuror is only demonstrating his incredible sleight of hand—defying us to discover how he does his tricks. But they *are* tricks. We all know that the lady was not really being sawn in half—logic convinces us of that—but this knowledge does not stop us enjoying the ghastly illusion. We are dealing in illusions, not delusions.

If through fear someone is unable to make his part of this agreement, it is important to understand why.

Some people are afraid to put their hands *inside* a puppet. There are people I have met who come forward at shows to touch the crocodile puppet, but who when offered the puppet to actually work draw back in horror at the prospect of seeing their own hand disappearing inside it. The crocodile might seem an obvious puppet to cause fear—but the same behaviour has been repeated with other puppets.

Suggestions:
Use a number of puppets which are being *visibly* manipulated.

> Wooden spoon puppets
> Finger puppets
> Rod puppets
> Plastic bag puppets.

These puppets can be worked without the hand disappearing. The plastic bag puppet is especially useful, because although the hand does go into the glove it never goes out of sight. Gradually the glove may be covered in self-adhesive shapes until there is no longer any sight of the hand inside. The young puppeteer must do this himself, and should also be encouraged to peep through the gaps to see his hand "still there".

Use a puppet such as Ted—remember he is worked by rods—and work him to music. Get alongside the child yourself, perhaps with others, too, to make a friendly group.

Use Tubby—ask the child to work the head rod while you work the hands. You have to work very closely together, so be prepared to touch and embrace the child and try to achieve eye contact. Close body contact could be reassuring to the child and give him confidence.

Use the SIMON puppet—build him up piece by piece. The child achieves control by actually building the puppet before playing with him.

When possible, work in front of a mirror. This could be frightening, because the mirror image may seem to separate the child from himself. "Who is it there? Me? Another person? If I am in there where is the me that was here? How come someone is there that looks like me?"

Work only with a small mirror at first and then go on to working with a full-sized mirror. Show only the puppet in the mirror, and then later go on to show the whole person with the puppet.

Another reason for disliking puppets may simply be that there are too many other things to be doing. And that is an excellent thought. Puppetry is only one of the performing arts, and if there are other things going on, and we have musicians,

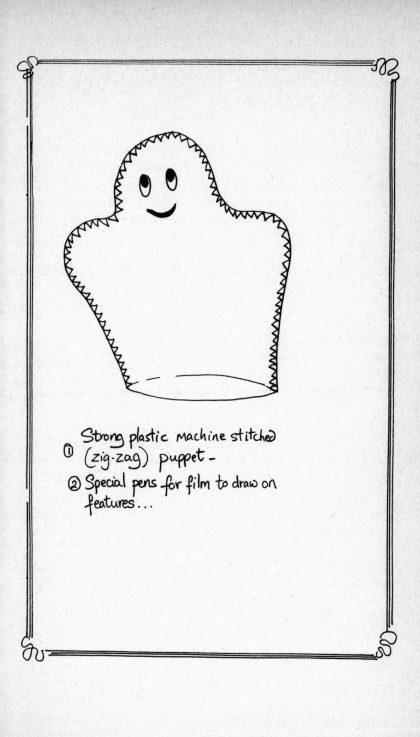

① Strong plastic machine stitched (zig-zag) puppet -

② Special pens for film to draw on features...

singers, and actors too who are also mentally handicapped people, then puppetry is just one of the options, which of course, is the way things should be.

And finally a story—a true story. I went along to the school for the weekly session on puppets with some physically handicapped children. Along the corridor I met Peggy—dragging herself along by the hand-rail. Peggy had been normal when born, but when she was about two her father battered her and left her paralysed down one side of her body and intellectually impaired. Now at thirteen a large over-developed teenager, it was unusual to see her out of her wheelchair. She told me about *Heidi* on television—about the girl in the wheelchair who had jumped out and started to walk again. Watching Peggy who was coming a poor second to a miracle, I saw the power of her imagination taking her on to ever greater heights: she was determined to do better.

A generous, kind child, very open to anything new, she was an enthusiastic puppeteer from the very beginning. She decided to use a sleeve puppet, and was keen to put it on to her bad hand—the one which was clutched into a fist at her side all the time. Through the rehearsals it seemed unlikely she would be able to lift her arm high enough for the audience to see the puppet. The day of the show came along. The children were very excited, and when friends and staff were all sitting quietly we began. I was backstage—behind the screen, helping the children and pushing wheelchairs into place—when Peggy's teacher came round to me in great agitation: "Look! Look at Peggy's arm." The swan puppet was stretching and bowing its beautiful neck in a wonderfully graceful movement. Was it really the clumsy handicapped teenager working that puppet? It was.

The excitement of performing, of having all those friends and staff out there—not waiting for anything else—but come specially for *their* show, the tension, the anticipation had completely overridden the effect of paralysis. There were people out there who were waiting for her to say what she had to say—to see her work her puppet . . .

No—there is no permanent cure. Even though a puppet

show can be a highlight in the life of a handicapped person like Peggy, the lights are in fact dimming. Puppet shows are not reality. As art they might represent a view on reality, they are the product of the potential which everyone like Peggy has. But even in those moments when a damaged limb can appear to work normally, the reality is that in the real world Peggy is viewed as having very little potential.

After a show in a theatre the auditorium empties and in my kind of show the house is left untidy. The wheelchairs have all gone, the lame have been led out, some seats are on their sides and the echoes of voices have died away. Often I get out quickly so that I'm not alone in the house; but sometimes I'll stop for a few seconds and my memory will fill with ghosts of sounds and movements from the show and audience: Lisa saying ''Flower'', David creeping forward—the look of rapture on the blind lady's face.

Resource List

SUPPLIERS OF MATERIALS

FIBREGLASS, CASTING PLASTER, RESINS, CARVING TOOLS, VICES etc: Alex Tiranti and Sons, 21 Goodge Place, London W1. Tel: 01-636 8565.

CARPENTRY TOOLS (extensive range): Parry and Sons, 329 Old Street, London EC1. Tel: 01-739 9422.

GLUES AND WOODWORKING TOOLS: Buck and Ryan, 101 Tottenham Court Road, London W1. Tel: 01-636 7475. Also: 55, Harrow Road, London W2. Tel: 01-723 6534.

JELUTONG AND WOODS FOR CARVING: William Bloore, 57 South Lambeth Road, London SW8. Tel: 01-735 7171.

COLOURED/STRIPED CANVAS (and fireproof gauze): Russell and Chapple Ltd., 23 Monmouth Street, London WC2. Tel: 01-836 7521.

(Canvas only) C. Hayward, 113 Nathan Way, Woolwich, London SE28. Tel: 01-854 3422.

SPONGE (FOAM) (all grades): Pentonville Rubber Co., 50/52 Pentonville Road, London N1. Tel: 01-837 0283.

POLYTHENE: Transatlantic Plastics, Surbiton, Surrey. Tel: 01-399 5271.

LATEX: D. B. Shipping Co. (Macadam & Co.) Monument House, Monument Street, London EC1. Tel: 01-626 8634.

CELASTIC: The Luck Counter Co., Spencer Street, Oadby, Leicester LE2 4DP. Tel: Leicester 713276/7. Also the Puppet Centre 01-228 5335.

FELT: The Felt Shop, 34 Granville Street, London EC1. Tel: 01-405 6215.

"RAWLPLUG" PLASTIC WOOD; C. Brewer & Sons, 327 Putney Bridge Road, London SW15. Tel: 01-788 9335, and most ironmongers, in small quantities.

ACETONE: Strand Glass Co., 524 High Street, Ilford, Essex. Tel: 01-599 8228/8238 (also fibreglass).

POLYSTYRENE AND FIBREGLASS: Adrian Merchant Ltd., Chesnut Grove, New Malden, Surrey. Tel: 01-942 9282.

GLITTER: Ells and Farrier Ltd., Bead Merchants, 5 Princes Street (off Regent Street), London W1. Tel: 01-629 9964.

PAINTS (and specialist artists material only); Michael J. Putman, 151 Lavender Hill, London SW11. Tel: 01-228 9087.

PAINTS (Theatre paints and materials): Brodie and Middleton Ltd., 79 Long Acre, London WC1. Tel: 01-836 3289.

THEATRICAL FABRICS: Borovick Fabrics Ltd., 16 Berwick Street, London W1. Tel: 01-437 2180.

TARLATAN AND SCRIM: Michael Putman, 151 Lavender Hill, London SW11. Tel: 01-228 9087.

THEATRE EFFECTS: (Flash powder etc): Theatrescene Armoury Ltd. 12/13 Henrietta Street, London W1. Tel: 01-240 2116/2231.

NOISE MAKERS (bird pipes, sirens, etc.): The Rhythm Box, 5 Denmark Street, London WC2. Tel: 01-240 3856.

DECORATIVE PAPERS: Paper Chase, 167 Fulham Road, London SW1. Tel: 01-589 7873, and 213 Tottenham Court Road, Tel: 01-580 8496.

SWAZZLES AND VENTRILOQUISM: L. Davenport and Co., 51 Great Russell Street, London WC1. Tel: 01-405 8524.

SUPREME MAGIC CO., 64 High Street, Bideford, Devon. Tel: 023 72 3625.

ULTRA-VIOLET LIGHTING TUBES: Service Trading Company, 9 Little Newport Street, Leicester Square, London WC2H 7J. Tel: 01-437 0576.

For people in the North

RUBBER PRODUCTS: Chapel Works, Ashley Road, Leeds 9. Another note about sponge (foam)—I have often managed to get it easily from market stalls and firms making furniture where they have offcuts.

Expanded polystyrene I get from shops selling large electrical goods—televisions and freezers. Fine grade polystyrene foam is used for pre-formed packaging.

Futurist Theatrical Hire Ltd., Blakeridge Lane, Batley, West Yorks. For lighting, acetates and special effects equipment.

Please join the Puppet Centre Trust—for details of courses, shows, lectures. At the Battersea Arts Centre the Trust have facilities comprising office, library, workshop, and exhibition space. The Education and Therapy unit will keep you in touch with events and give details about shows for handicapped people. They have a fine collection of puppetry books on sale: The Puppet Centre, Battersea Town Hall, London SW11. Tel: 01-228 5335.

Charig Puppets can make some of the puppets illustrated and used throughout the publication: 89 Skipton Road, Harrogate HG1 4LF. Tel. 0423 66138.

FURTHER READING

These are some of the books I have found useful in my work:
Music and Imagination, Aaron Copland, New English Library, 1952.
Art needs no justification, H. R. Rookmaker, Inter-Varsity Press, 1978.
Therapy in Music for Handicapped Children, Paul Nordoff and Clive Robbins, Victor Gollancz, 1971.
Developmental Art Therapy, Geraldine H. Williams and Mary M. Wood, University Park Press, 1977.
The World of Puppets, Rene Simmen, Phaidon.
Shadow Puppets, Shadow Theatres and Shadow Films, Lotte Reiniger, Play, Inc., Boston 1975.
The Know How Book of Puppets, Violet Philpott and Mary Jean McNeil, Usborne Publishing Ltd., 1975.
The Complete Book of Puppetry, David Currell, Pitman, 1974.
Puppets for Dreaming and Scheming; Judy Sims, Early Stages, California, 1978.
Puppetry Today, Helen Binyon, Studio Vista, 1966.
Puppets and Therapy, A. R. Philpott, Educational Puppetry Association (Puppet Centre Trust), Battersea Town Hall, Lavender Hill, London SW11.

Index